Lower Your BLOOD PRESSURE Naturally

Drop Pounds and Slash Your Blood Pressure in **6 Weeks** Without Drugs

Sari Harrar
and the Editors of **Prevention**
with Suzanne Steinbaum, DO

RODALE.

© 2014 by Rodale Inc.
Photographs © 2014 by Rodale Inc.

All rights reserved. No part of this publication may be reproduced or transmitted in any form or by any means, electronic or mechanical, including photocopying, recording, or any other information storage and retrieval system, without the written permission of the publisher.

Rodale books may be purchased for business or promotional use or for special sales. For information, please write to:
Special Markets Department, Rodale Inc., 733 Third Avenue, New York, NY 10017

Prevention is a registered trademark of Rodale Inc.

Printed in the United States of America
Rodale Inc. makes every effort to use acid-free ∞, recycled paper ♲.

Photographs by Mitch Mandel/Rodale Images

Book design by Elizabeth Neal

Library of Congress Cataloging-in-Publication Data is on file with the publisher.

ISBN 978-1-62336-234-8 hardcover

Distributed to the trade by Macmillan

2   4   6   8   10   9   7   5   3   1   hardcover

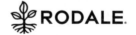

We inspire and enable people to improve their lives and the world around them.
rodalebooks.com

Contents

Part IV: More Tools

Acknowledgments

With deep appreciation to Dr. Suzanne Steinbaum for her passion, deep knowledge, humor, and down-to-earth, do-it-yourself savvy about healthy, natural blood pressure control; to Trisha Calvo and Sarah Pelz, our patient, insightful, and good-humored editors; to Stephanie Clarke and Willow Jarosh of C&J Nutrition for developing a delicious, mineral-packed eating plan and answering countless questions; to Jess Fromm for gracefully managing a million details; to *Prevention*'s fitness director, Jenna Bergen, for designing the book's innovative fitness plan and to Bari Lieberman, *Prevention*'s senior associate fitness director, for demonstrating it; and to Hope Clarke, Elizabeth Neal, Wendy Gable, Susan Hindman, and Michelle Janowitz for creating this powerful and beautiful book.

Special thanks to our intrepid test panelists who changed their daily lives for 6 weeks to test the plan, overcoming all sorts of obstacles along the way, from broken arms and family medical emergencies to getting up early to exercise.

Part I

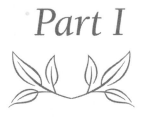

Better Blood Pressure and a Slimmer You!

CHAPTER 1

The Natural Solution for High Blood Pressure

How's your blood pressure?

It's an urgent question no man or woman can afford to ignore. Living with high blood pressure is like having an invisible, raging river speeding through your arteries day and night. It damages artery walls, and it can harm almost every organ in your body. And living with this "raging river" in your arteries is just downright dangerous.

High blood pressure has been dubbed "the silent killer" because it often has no warning signs or symptoms. It is also linked to many other health complications: It doubles your odds for a heart attack, raises your risk for a stroke fourfold,[1] and increases your chances for everything from dementia and kidney failure to vision loss, sexual dysfunction, and even weak bones. Seventy percent of people who have had a heart attack or stroke, it turns out, have high blood pressure. It can steal 5 years from your life.[2] And it is the number one cause of preventable, heart-related deaths in America.[3]

The shocker? Almost all of us have high blood pressure or are at high risk for developing it. Two-thirds of Americans have hypertension (a blood pressure reading of 140/90 or higher) or prehypertension (a higher-than-healthy reading between 120/80 and 139/89). And if you're among the one in three with healthy blood pressure levels, hypertension may very well be in your future. Your lifetime risk for developing this invisible, unfelt threat is a whopping 90 percent. By age 60, 50 percent of us will have high blood pressure, and most of the time it is due to our lifestyle choices.

However, more Americans than ever before are aware of high blood pressure and trying to do something about it. The number of people whose BP (shorthand for "blood pressure," which you'll see throughout this book) is being treated doubled between 1988 and 2008. Hypertension is now the most frequently diagnosed health condition that turns up in the 1 billion visits we make to our doctors each year,[4] and it is the specific reason for 39 million of those appointments.[5] We spend nearly $70 billion trying to take care of it.[6]

But there's still a huge and frustrating gap. Half of the 78 million women and men with high blood pressure don't have it under control.[7] And just one in three of the 70 million with prehypertension do. The reasons?

Medication alone isn't the answer. Taking one, two, or even three different drugs for high blood pressure often cannot overcome the everyday factors that cause high BP and conspire to drive it higher and higher.

Making the wrong lifestyle changes can lead you to believe that do-it-yourself strategies don't work. If you've ever tried to drop a few pounds or cut out a little salt to lower your BP, only to see your numbers barely budge, you know what we're talking about.

There's a better way to lower your blood pressure—effectively, naturally, and often without adding more drugs or increasing the dose of current medications. It's the synergistic, breakthrough approach in this book we created with the help of Suzanne Steinbaum, DO, a leading cardiologist and the director of Women and Heart Disease at Lenox Hill Hospital in New York City. It helped our test panelists, all of whom started the 6-week program with high blood pressure, lower their numbers significantly and, as a result, slash their risk for heart attacks, strokes, and all of hypertension's other life-altering consequences.

Real Results

Lower Your Blood Pressure Naturally is the only plan that attacks the root causes of high blood pressure on all fronts with eight proven, drug-free strategies. The lifestyle changes you'll make on this plan are proven to work individually, but emerging research shows that combining them increases their pressure-lowering power.

That's the magic of synergy. But it's not the only magic in this plan. Every step is easy and convenient, so that you can benefit from pressure-lowering synergy on your craziest, busiest days and make this 6-week plan a permanent part of your life.

Our test panelists are the proof. When our seven volunteers with high blood pressure—women and men ages 26 to 75—followed the Lower Your Blood Pressure Naturally plan for 6 weeks, the results were spectacular. Everyone reduced their blood pressure, lowering systolic blood pressure (the top number in a BP reading) by as much as 30 points and diastolic blood pressure (the bottom number) by as much as 17 points. Several panelists taking blood pressure drugs without much success were finally able to reach healthy levels. Two even worked with their doctors to reduce their medications.

In fact, Dr. Steinbaum finds that the effects of lifestyle changes on lowering blood pressure are powerful. "I am often asked by patients if going on blood pressure medication is a life sentence. I always explain that someone who is determined to come off medication can do so. Medication is not forever if you commit to making lifestyle changes that alter your body's physiology. This synergistic plan demonstrates this truth and shows you how it actually can be done," she explains.

In addition, test panelists dropped up to 14.4 pounds and trimmed their waistlines by as much as 5¼ inches. They bought new clothes, found they could button pants that had grown too tight, slipped into outfits that had been in mothballs since college, and basked in the glow of compliments from family, friends, and coworkers.

You'll hear firsthand how well this program worked for our test panelists in their profiles throughout this book, but here's a sneak peek at their stories.

- **"I've gone from a size 12 to a size 10 and sometimes even wear a size 8.** My boss and my husband both say they can't believe the difference," says Penny Boos, 55. Even better: Penny, who survived a heart attack in 2012, reduced her blood pressure from 150/80—a reading that put her into the hypertensive category—to a healthy 124/67, which significantly lowers her risk for heart attacks and strokes.

- **"When I started seeing results, I was really amazed,"** says Chris Colbaugh, 32, who lost 8.4 pounds and lowered his blood pressure enough to reduce his medication. "All I had to do was change my diet, exercise, and learn to meditate. It was that simple. A lot of people try crazy diets, and these really aren't necessary. You just need to cut back on sodium and get plenty of calcium, magnesium, and potassium."

- **"Getting my weight below 200 was an absolute triumph,"** says Tom Colbaugh, 59, who lost $14\frac{1}{2}$ pounds and reduced his blood pressure from 193/82 to 163/65 in 4 weeks. Tom, who is Chris's father, stuck with the plan for a total of 10 weeks, losing 20 pounds in all and further reducing his blood pressure to a healthy 127/57. "I haven't been this weight in 20 years, and I haven't had my blood pressure under control this good for a long time. I'm planning to do this forever."

- **"I never thought it would be possible to take off the extra weight,"** especially the fat around my midsection that has been creeping on over the past few years," noted Anita Hirsch, 75, who lost 10.6 pounds and reduced her blood pressure from 145/80 to 116/71 in 6 weeks. "It was really gratifying to lose stomach fat. It's the bad kind that causes heart problems."

- **"It's a safe, natural way for me to control my blood pressure,"** says David Oblas, 28, who lowered his BP from a high of 145/89 to a healthy 119/73 in 6 weeks. "Throughout my life, doctors have tried to get me to go on some type of blood pressure medication, and I always refused, knowing that there was likely a safer and healthier way."

Eight Synergistic Strategies

How did they do it? With the same eight strategies you'll deploy daily on this plan. Here they are.

1. **Eat less salt, but never have a bland meal.** This plan lowers your intake of sodium—a proven blood pressure booster—to a healthy, moderate amount: 2,300 milligrams per day. That's low enough to help reverse high blood pressure, but not so low that you're stuck eating tasteless food. You'll learn how to use a few grains of salt to intensify flavor and how to create our five low-salt and no-salt spice blends that enhance the taste of food even

more. Don't believe what the media say about salt being "safe" or low-sodium diets being problematic (more on this in Chapter 3). Salt raises blood pressure by increasing the fluid level in your blood, and in many people, especially African Americans, salt in excess is correlated with hypertension, secondary to poor diets that are filled with salt. The truth is, most Americans eat too much of this stuff, most of it from packaged, processed, and restaurant foods.

2. **Enjoy mineral-packed meals that regulate blood pressure naturally.** Most of us don't get nearly enough calcium, magnesium, and potassium from food, which is the best source of these important, pressure-controlling minerals. More and more research is showing that healthy BP control relies on getting twice as much potassium as sodium every day, yet just 2 percent of us hit that ratio. On this plan, you'll get 1,200 milligrams of calcium, 4,700 milligrams of potassium, and 420 milligrams of magnesium every day. In Phase 1, all of the meals are built around 13 Power Foods that deliver big doses of these minerals. Several test panelists told us their blood pressure began moving in a healthy direction within the first week; we suspect that a better mineral balance is a big reason. In Phase 2, you'll eat a wide variety of foods that provide these key nutrients.

3. **Fit in a pressure-lowering interval walk.** You'll do a 20-minute interval walk 3 days a week. Alternating between fast and moderate walking speeds can actually lower BP better than sticking with just a steady pace. On other days, you will walk at a steady pace (as a break from interval walks) but can break it up into two or three shorter walks a day—a time-saver that actually keeps your BP lower, longer.

4. **Strength-train twice a week.** Our six-move routine takes just 15 minutes yet works every muscle group. Strength training helps you lose weight, which itself lowers blood pressure. Anyone can do this easy routine. By choosing the right weights for you, it's safe and effective for beginners and experienced exercisers. Strength training is one of the "blood pressure bonuses" you'll enjoy daily on the plan.

5. **Do yoga four times a week.** You will alternate between yoga and strength training to fit in your daily blood pressure bonus. On yoga days, your choices are an invigorating morning session or a relaxing restorative routine at the end of your day. Each takes just 15 minutes and includes easy moves and modifications so it's right for everyone. Yoga decreases stress and dials down your nervous system's fight-or-flight response, reducing stress hormone levels that boost blood pressure by tightening arteries.

6. **Lose weight.** You'll lose pounds, inches, and belly fat (like our test panelists did!) without counting calories. And trimming excess weight reduces blood pressure. It gives your heart a break, lessens the inflammation that contributes to high blood pressure, and even takes pressure off your kidneys, which play a big part in BP control.

7. **Tame tension in 5 minutes.** You will learn to relax with a soothing 5-minute daily meditation. This do-anywhere, do-anytime technique can help shut down stress, thereby easing blood pressure. Test panelists told us they found themselves using their breath to calm down whenever they felt tense.

8. **Track your blood pressure.** Research shows that keeping tabs on your blood pressure can help you reduce it by a few points. Knowing your numbers will help you stay accountable. Seeing results will inspire you to keep going strong! Our test panelists used inexpensive home blood pressure monitors. You can, too. Or take advantage of free blood pressure checks in your community to stay on top of your numbers between doctor visits.

Fast, Delicious Meals; Smoothies; and Desserts

How about waking up to a creamy smoothie, a bowl of hot cereal topped with sweet peaches, or eggs and hash browns? Or serving your family a luscious pork tenderloin for Sunday dinner, along with garlic-seasoned broccoli and quinoa (a nutty, fast-cooking whole grain)? Or treating yourself (and your significant other and kids) to ice cream and a cookie, chocolate–peanut butter frozen yogurt, or a cup of hot cocoa in the evening? All the while knowing that the food you're enjoying is designed by Mother Nature to promote healthy blood pressure levels? (The healthiest foods don't come in packages with ingredients that you cannot pronounce; they come in their original packaging from nature.)

That's the rationale behind our eating plan. Our test panelists loved the flexibility and the great food. They took it to work, savored it on road trips, and served it to guests and visiting family. And they stuck to the plan easily at picnics, parties, and when there was literally no time to cook after long workdays or during family emergencies. When they saw how the plan's moderate-sodium, mineral-packed foods reduced their blood pressure, they loved it even more.

Our eating plan was developed by registered dietitians Willow Jarosh and Stephanie Clarke, nutrition experts who know the hard science behind food's effects on the human body and how to translate it into tasty, fun, sumptuous meals that will keep you (and your family) satisfied. When we asked them to turn the latest nutritional knowledge about natural blood pressure control into an eating plan, we were amazed by the versatility and creativity of their menus and recipes. The eating plan features:

- **13 Power Foods.** For the first week of the plan, you'll follow our Phase 1 jump-start menu that uses just 13 mineral-packed foods and a few basic kitchen staples to create breakfasts, lunches, dinners, and a daily Power Mineral Smoothie. Each Power Food is a rich source of at least two of our three Power Minerals: calcium, magnesium, and potassium. And working with just 13 ingredients makes grocery shopping a breeze. You'll discover plenty of new ways to fit these important foods into your meals, giving you Power Food expertise that will help you keep your mineral intake high once the plan ends. Our 13 Power Foods are: avocados, bananas, broccoli, kale, kiwifruit, peaches (or nectarines), pork tenderloin, quinoa, red bell peppers, sweet potatoes, tilapia, white beans, and fat-free yogurt. More on these later!

- **Four meals a day.** Beginning with Phase 1 and continuing through Phase 2, you'll choose four meals a day from our selection of delicious breakfast, lunch, and dinner options. Test panelists told us they sometimes couldn't eat all the meals! (Foods that are filled with nutrients are more satiating. Gradually, the body only craves foods that are healthy and can't quite tolerate those that are not. After following the plan, many test panelists found restaurant foods too salty to enjoy!) Packed with high-satisfaction foods loaded with fiber, good fat, and lean protein, these meals are designed for weight loss, yet you never have to count calories. Hearty, tasty choices include breakfast options like Cheesy Potato Hash Topped with an Egg (page 111) and Blueberries and Cream Protein Pancakes (page 107); fast lunches like the Avocado, Provolone, Hummus, Cucumber, and Tomato Sandwich (page 131); and dinner favorites like Orange-Ginger Halibut (page 115), Fiesta Shrimp Tacos (page 114), Garlic-Ginger Tofu Stir-Fry (page 116), and Dukkah-Spiced Pork Tenderloin with Broccoli and Quinoa (page 96).

- **A Power Mineral Smoothie or Power Mineral Dessert every day in Phase 2.** In addition to your four daily meals, help yourself to a smoothie or dessert every day in Weeks 2 through 6. These tasty additions bump up your mineral intake and provide pressure-pampering fiber and (yes!) even some chocolate. How about Peanut Butter–Banana Frozen Yogurt (page 129), Double-Dark Hot Chocolate (page 128), a Peach-Almond Ice Cream Cup (page 127), or a Berries and Cream Smoothie (page 126)?

- **Flavorful spice blends and a better way to use your saltshaker.** Never dull, the food you'll enjoy on this plan is well seasoned. You'll find directions starting on page 84 for whipping up our five spice blends: Tex-Mex, Italian, Indian, a BBQ rub, and intriguing Dukkah, a Middle Eastern seasoning mix that's delicious on everything. You'll also discover the best way to use small amounts of salt for maximum flavor without the pressure-boosting effect: Research shows that a few grains on ready-to-serve food is all you need.

Start Today!

High blood pressure is a serious health condition that is so out of control in America that the Centers for Disease Control and Prevention recently declared it "public health enemy number two," right behind smoking.[8] Medicine helps. But there's plenty more you can do to lower your numbers naturally and effectively with the plan in this book.

Taking care of your blood pressure is one of the most powerful ways you can protect your health. Research shows that reducing high levels can slash your chances of having a stroke by 35 to 40 percent, lower your odds for a heart attack by 20 to 25 percent, and shrink your risk for heart failure by 50 percent.[9]

Get started by finding out what your blood pressure is and discussing this plan with your doctor if your levels are high. If you take high blood pressure medications, continue to do so. Never stop or change a dose on your own. (Test panelists who reduced their doses did so after monitoring their pressure levels daily and working with their doctors to make changes.) This plan can help you improve your numbers and the health of your cardiovascular system whether you use hypertension medications or not.

Success Story: *Chris Colbaugh*

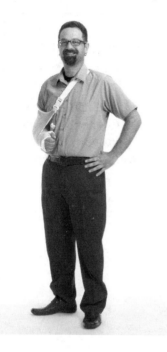

AGE: 32

HEIGHT: 5'11"

BLOOD PRESSURE IMPROVEMENT:
Chris kept his blood pressure at
healthy levels while reducing his blood
pressure medication.

POUNDS LOST: 8.4

"My blood pressure hasn't been this low
since high school," says Chris. "My doctor is really impressed. He says if I lose a
few more pounds, I may not need medication at all."

An avid bicyclist and skier, Chris
says plenty of exercise helped him keep
his blood pressure in check through his
twenties, until a series of accidents
forced him to cut back. "I hurt my neck,
my knee, my arm," he explains. "It was kind of a downward spiral. I was
still active, but not as much. And with the blood pressure problems in my
family, I'm not surprised it caught up to me, too."

Chris reorganized his grocery shopping routine before starting the eating plan. "I didn't eat like this at all before. It was a total 180-degree rever-
sal. Between my work schedule and living alone, my diet wasn't so great,"
he says. "On the plan, I had to learn how to get all my food prepped. And I
had to learn to like green veggies. I found out I do like broccoli and baby
spinach. And I eat a lot more sweet potatoes than white potatoes these
days."

A breakfast fan, Chris would have a smoothie when he woke up and
then one of his favorites—like the oat-based pancakes (page 107) in Phase
2 or the Open-Faced Avocado-Mozzarella Egg Sandwich (page 108)—an
hour or so later. "I can't eat a big meal first thing in the morning," he
explains. He would then pack up a dinner to take to his job as a machinist.
"If I had one break, I'd eat a big meal that combined two of the meals from

the plan. If I had two breaks, I'd eat two meals. There are so many food options on this plan, so I always had plenty to eat. The fast, easy sandwiches were good for me to put together quickly and take to work."

Losing 8 pounds as well as an inch from his waist means Chris's clothes are no longer snug. "I've been the same size since high school," he says. "All my pants were starting to get a little tight, but now the buttons are working just fine."

Chris discovered that the daily 5-minute meditation made him more aware of his stress level and better able to ease it at any time of day. "Sitting there and controlling my breathing was the best part of the workout," he says. "If I felt my pulse go up when I was tense, I could bring it back down naturally. I would do the meditation for 5 to 10 minutes before I went to sleep. And I would sleep much better. If you focus on your breathing, you get out of your head and into your body. It helps me with everything else I do."

He also discovered how good yoga feels. "It stretches me out. I love the feeling," he says. "My body just wants to keep doing it. Overall, when everything came together and I started to get results, I got this big smile on my face. The plan brings together all of the research and it works. I feel better."

CHAPTER 2

The Hidden High Blood Pressure Crisis

Imagine a sparkling stream peacefully meandering through a summer meadow. Then, a sudden downpour changes the scene. The placid brook is now a raging torrent, tearing at its banks with the force of a water cannon.

Now imagine this happening inside your body. As unbelievable as it may sound, it is a dangerous reality. You can't feel or see this health-wrecker, but high blood pressure causes or contributes to more than 348,000 deaths a year in the United States.[1]

Tackling high blood pressure is crucial. Heart health experts consider it one of the chief risk factors for heart disease (America's number one killer) and stroke (America's number three killer and number one cause of disabilities). Some go further, calling it *the* most important and controllable risk factor. But that's the empowering news: You can be the boss of your blood pressure by making simple lifestyle changes and, if needed, by taking pressure-lowering medications. The best lifestyle approach is the one touted in this book, which attacks the root causes of rising BP with eight proven, synergistic strategies.

But first, let's get down to basics: understanding high blood pressure by the numbers.

Blood pressure is the force of blood against the inner walls of your arteries. Since you cannot see or feel most blood pressure changes, knowing your numbers—and what they mean—is the only way to be sure your BP is behaving.

Many of us only think about our blood pressure when a doctor, nurse, or other health care practitioner wraps that thick cuff around our upper arm. You know the drill. You rush into the examining room, perch on the table, and roll up your sleeve. The practitioner inflates the cuff until it's uncomfortably snug, then carefully monitors a dial, gauge, or digital display. The silence in the room is broken only by the *hiss!* of the cuff deflating. You long to ask, "Well, how's my blood pressure?" But you don't dare break the silence during this ritual.

After the latest numbers are recorded in your chart, we hope you and your doctor do break the silence about high blood pressure. Too often, this important health indicator doesn't get the attention it deserves. Your doctor may simply give you an overview: "It's okay" or "It's a little high, let's watch that" or "It's time to increase your medication." Then again, you may be given plenty of information, but in the bustle of the typical 18-minute medical appointment, you might forget the details. Studies show that doctors and their patients both share responsibility for gaps in BP knowledge and control.

If you're not sure about your numbers, you're not alone. In one new study that quizzed people with high blood pressure about their condition, 1 in 12 didn't know their current levels. Half didn't know what their ideal blood pressure levels should even be.[2]

Let's change that right away. As you begin the Lower Your Blood Pressure Naturally plan, we want you to know your current BP numbers. We also want you to recheck them regularly so you can track changes. Get a current

---

Stop! What's Your BP?

Do you know your blood pressure numbers? If so, take a moment to write them down as your starting point on page 254. If not, find out soon (like today). It's the important first step to lowering your blood pressure naturally.

BP reading by visiting your doctor's office, by getting a free BP check in your community, or by using that blood pressure testing machine at the drugstore.

Regular home checks with an inexpensive monitor plus doctor check-ins is emerging as the gold standard for better blood pressure control. (That's how our test panelists kept current on their BP changes.) You'll feel motivated as you see your numbers improve. And if you use blood pressure drugs, you'll partner with your doctor to keep your doses fine-tuned. (If you take medication, follow the directions in Chapter 6 for working with your doctor. Do not change a dose or a drug on your own.)

What *Over* Huh? *Decode Your Numbers*

Blood pressure is always expressed as two numbers. Written down, they're separated by a slash, like 119/79 or 140/90. Read aloud, the slash becomes

---

Blast from the Past: The First Blood Pressure Monitor

A German scientist named Samuel Siegfried Karl Ritter von Basch invented the world's first BP monitor in 1861. It was a bulky contraption that strapped to the wrist and involved a water-filled rubber bulb, tubing, and a mercury-filled gauge. Modern monitors are easier to use and more accurate, but 21st-century BP checks carry these echoes from history.

MM HG: These letters often appear after blood pressure numbers (such as 118/77 mm Hg). They're an abbreviation for "millimeters of mercury," the unit of measurement used for BP readings.

SPHYGMOMANOMETER: The original name for a blood pressure monitor, this tongue twister is still found in medical-supply catalogs and on the packages of some monitors. Pronounced "SFIG-mo-ma-nom-e-ter," it comes from the Greek words *sphygmo* (pulse), *manos* ("thin," referring to the tube of mercury), and *meter* (measure).

---

the word *over*, like 118 over 76, or 155 over 82. The first or top number, always the higher of the two, is systolic blood pressure. That's the force of blood in your arteries during a heartbeat. The second or bottom number, always the lower of the two, is diastolic blood pressure. That's the force of blood against artery walls between heartbeats.

Both numbers are important. You can have prehypertension or hypertension if just one is elevated, for example. In the past, doctors focused more on controlling diastolic blood pressure. Old thinking was that an occasional spike in systolic pressure was normal and nonthreatening.

Not now. New medical thinking calls for paying particular attention to systolic blood pressure in people older than 50. It tends to rise with age due to stiffening of arteries and plaque buildup in artery walls (atherosclerosis). Elevated systolic pressure is a potent risk factor for heart disease, and it can be harder to control than diastolic pressure as we age.

The picture is slightly different for some younger people. About 40 percent of those under age 40 and 30 percent between ages 40 and 50 with high blood pressure only have elevated diastolic pressure. Experts now know that this also boosts risk for heart problems, especially if other risk factors are present, such as high cholesterol, diabetes, being overweight, or a history of smoking. Younger people with high diastolic pressure are also at risk for high systolic pressure in the long run.

The bottom line for all ages: It's important to get both numbers down to healthy levels.[3]

Can You Go *Too* Low?

Your blood pressure is considered low if the top number falls below 90 or the second falls below 60. You may feel dizzy or light-headed, especially when you get up from a chair or bed; you may also have a headache or feel tired. If you feel this way, use your blood pressure monitor to check your BP. If it's low, have a little salt—some salty nuts or pretzels or salt some vegetables—washed down with a glass of water. This can increase your blood pressure. If symptoms persist or return, call your doctor.

Blood pressure levels are divided into five categories by the American Heart Association.

CATEGORY	SYSTOLIC MM HG (UPPER #)	DIASTOLIC MM HG (LOWER #)
Normal	less than 120	and less than 80
Prehypertension	120–139	or 80–89
High Blood Pressure (Hypertension) Stage 1	140–159	or 90–99
High Blood Pressure (Hypertension) Stage 2	160 or higher	or 100 or higher
Hypertensive Crisis (emergency care needed)	higher than 180	or higher than 110

The View from Inside: Blood Pressure 101

Healthy BP is always changing. It naturally rises with every heartbeat and falls between beats. It also speeds up and slows down to meet your ever-changing needs. Under stress? Racing across the parking lot to get to work on time? Your blood pressure will increase in order to boost the supply of oxygen to your muscles, brain, organs, and other body tissues. Petting the dog? Rocking a baby to sleep or cuddling serenely with your sweetheart? When you're relaxed, blood pressure falls.

Your biological clock also tells your BP when to rise and fall. Blood pressure is naturally lowest at night when you're sleeping. It surges upward in the early morning before you wake up, continues to rise until midmorning, and then eases back down.[4] By the time you're back in bed asleep, it may have dropped 15 to 25 percent from its highest daytime point. In people with high blood pressure, however, the night drops may be smaller and the morning spikes extra large, boosting the risk for morning strokes and heart attacks. In fact, high blood pressure only at night is a problem worth treating even if daytime levels are closer to the normal range.

Flatten Morning Surges and Get Your "Night Dip" Back

For up to 40 percent of people with high blood pressure, nighttime levels don't quite drop to the natural lows that give the heart and arteries a break. This raises the risk for heart attacks, strokes, and other damage. Reducing sodium and getting regular exercise—two features of the Lower Your Blood Pressure Naturally plan—can help you regain this important time-out. [5, 6]

Meanwhile, the natural morning rise in blood pressure may be extra large in people with hypertension, boosting the odds for morning heart attacks and strokes. Risk is especially high for people who smoke, consume excess alcohol,[7] and have diets that are extra salty.[8] Quitting smoking and cutting back on alcohol helps. Research also shows that a diet low in sodium and packed with pressure-lowering calcium, magnesium, and potassium—like the eating plan in this book—reduces morning surges while keeping your BP lower all day and all night.[9]

Your Blood Pressure Control Center

Behind the scenes, your body regulates blood pressure in three ingenious ways: by raising or lowering your heart rate; by relaxing or tightening your blood vessels; and by increasing or decreasing the amount of fluid in your bloodstream.

Your brain and kidneys run this show. If your blood pressure falls too low (for example, if you stand up too quickly after waking up in the morning), your brain may churn out neurotransmitters called catecholamines to tighten blood vessels and make your heart beat faster and harder. Under stress? Your brain may tell your adrenal glands to release epinephrine and norepinephrine, hormones that increase your heart rate as part of your body's ancient fight-or-flight response.

Your kidneys contribute to blood pressure regulation in profound ways. They can produce renin, a chemical that constricts blood vessels. And by releasing or absorbing fluid and sodium from your urine, they also boost or reduce the fluid level in your bloodstream.

When Pressure Rises

But blood pressure doesn't always stay within a healthy range. Many factors can override your body's natural, beautifully balanced system to push BP into the danger zone. Some—such as your age, your genes, and your racial heritage—are beyond your control. But most are within your power.

Most people with high blood pressure have a type called primary (or essential) hypertension. It isn't caused by a single, fixable, underlying problem like an overactive thyroid, a kidney disorder, off-balance hormones, or sleep apnea. In fact, top heart health doctors maintain that sometimes there's no identifiable cause for primary hypertension. Sounds crazy, doesn't it? With more than 368,000 high blood pressure studies published in medical journals since 1908 and nearly 1 billion people around the world living with hypertension, can medical science really shrug its shoulders and say, "Well, we just don't know why"?

It turns out this is true, but it's not the whole truth. What experts really mean is that many factors contribute to primary hypertension, but it's nearly impossible to pinpoint which led to yours. Is it because your mom, grandfather, and four cousins all have high blood pressure? And how much of the blame should go to those 17 extra pounds, your high-stress job, or your penchant for fast-food tacos on Friday night?

Just don't ever misinterpret "We don't know why" as "There's nothing you can do." Solid scientific research has indeed nabbed the major culprits. And new studies show that for many people, lifestyle factors in your control are even more powerful than the factors you cannot change.

The top causes of high blood pressure that you can't control are:

Genes: Genes carry about 30 percent of the blame for hypertension, say Harvard Medical School researchers.[10] And researchers are discovering more and more genetic quirks that contribute to the extra risk. Most often, the culprit is actually a constellation of genes interacting with pressure-raising forces in your life such as weight, diet, or activity level.

Racial heritage: African Americans are more likely to develop hypertension than Caucasians. It starts earlier and can be more severe, substantially increasing the risk for kidney problems[11] and strokes.[12] Researchers suspect that genetics, plus factors in daily life, such as diet and exercise levels, may explain the risk.[13]

Aging: If you do not have hypertension by age 55 to 65, your risk for developing it is a whopping 90 percent say researchers with the landmark

Synergy Trumps the Biggest BP Risks

Think you can't overcome so-called uncontrollable high blood pressure risks, like your age or your family history? Here's proof that they're no match for the strategies you'll find in the Lower Your Blood Pressure Naturally plan.

Overcome aging: In a Johns Hopkins University study of 975 women and men ages 60 to 80 with hypertension, weight loss plus cutting back on salty foods (two components of our plan) helped 40 percent of participants lower their numbers enough to stop taking blood pressure medications.[14]

Reduce the effects of genetic risk: Genes don't necessarily have the final say. In a 2013 study from the Cardiovascular Institute of New Jersey at the University of Medicine and Dentistry of New Jersey-Robert Wood Johnson Medical School, people with genetic risk factors for hypertension lowered their numbers with weight loss and a reduced-sodium meal plan.[15]

Minimize inherited risks: African Americans are at higher risk for hypertension. When 412 women and men, 54 percent of whom were African American, reduced sodium and bumped up their intake of healthy foods containing calcium, magnesium, and potassium, they got big results. African American participants with hypertension lowered their systolic blood pressure by 10 points and diastolic pressure by 5 points.[16]

Framingham Heart Study.[17] By age 60, 50 percent of people will have high blood pressure. But diet, exercise, and stress reduction (the steps in this plan) can prevent you from becoming part of this 50 percent. While aging can stiffen arteries, it doesn't have to nudge your BP out of the safety zone or keep it elevated.

And the top causes of high blood pressure that you *can* control are:

Too much sodium: The average American downs 30 percent more sodium than is healthy, most of it hidden in packaged, processed, and restaurant foods. When your kidneys can't filter out all of the excess, it stays in your bloodstream along with surplus fluid, boosting blood volume and thereby increasing blood pressure. If your diet is also low in potassium (as most Americans' diets are), your kidneys hold on to extra sodium as they attempt to keep potassium levels in your body high. But that's not all. New Harvard Medical School research suggests high-sodium diets directly damage blood vessels, further elevating risk for high blood pressure.[18] Read more in Chapter 3 about why reducing sodium to moderate levels, as you will on this plan, is crucial despite what you may have seen in the media.

Not enough calcium, magnesium, and potassium: These minerals are critical to healthy blood pressure because they help your body keep sodium under control and help artery walls relax. Yet, as you'll discover in Chapter 4, most of us don't get enough of them from food, the most effective source for blood pressure control. At the same time, we overindulge in sodium, throwing off the natural mineral balance that promotes healthy blood pressure. The fix: This plan restores that balance by reducing sodium and delivering a full dose of the Power Minerals you need.

Extra pounds and extra belly fat: Body fat needs oxygen and fuel to survive, just like your muscles and organs. Extra fat prompts your heart to work harder, pumping blood faster and more forcefully. This boosts blood pressure. Excess belly fat, in particular, revs up blood pressure by releasing chemicals that constrict blood vessels. Researchers from the University of São Paulo in Brazil suspect that deep abdominal fat also squeezes the kidneys, prompting them to hold on to excess sodium.[19] The fix: Losing weight and belly fat is a powerful way to tame rising blood pressure, as our test panelists discovered. Research backs it up: In one study, people with prehypertension who lost just 4.4 pounds reduced their systolic blood pressure by 3.7 points and their diastolic pressure by 2.7 points. As a result, 42 percent of them returned to healthy blood pressure levels.[20]

No exercise: People who rarely exercise tend to have higher heart rates. That means your ticker has to work harder every time it contracts to pump blood through your circulatory system. This raises your blood pressure. Of course, skipping or skimping on exercise also boosts your odds for extra pounds. The fix: Short routines that make the most of your time and that are proven to do more to control blood pressure. On this plan, you'll discover the fat-burning, belly-fat-blasting benefits of interval walking and strength training. In just 30 to 45 minutes a day, you'll lose pounds and inches while giving your cardiovascular system the workout it needs to lower pressure naturally.

Chronic stress: Tense up and your body releases a cascade of hormones that can constrict blood vessels and increase your heart rate. In prehistoric times, your body's fight-or-flight response helped you outrun predators and stay safe. But modern stress assails us around the clock, contributing to higher BP. Studies show that meditation and yoga can assist in lowering blood pressure. The 5-minute breathing meditation and short yoga routines you'll find in this plan can bring new pressure-lowering serenity to your life.

Overindulging in alcohol: Ethanol—the alcohol in beer, wine, and hard liquors—relaxes arteries for moderate drinkers. This is one reason health groups say that up to one daily drink for women and two for men may lower heart risks for many people. Go higher, however, and everything changes. In a Harvard School of Public Health study of 14,892 people, women who had two to three drinks a day boosted high blood pressure risk 10 percent. Those who had four to five daily drinks increased risk 84 percent. Men's risk rose 29 percent for those having more than two daily drinks.[21] Alcohol may raise risk by altering body chemistry and activating the sympathetic nervous system in ways that tighten arteries, the researchers report. On this plan, you'll steer clear of alcohol for 6 weeks in order to keep calorie intake low.

Smoking: Your first cigarette of the day can temporarily raise systolic blood pressure by 20 points.[22] If you have mild hypertension, the combination of smoking and sipping coffee through the day can keep your blood

---

Secondary Hypertension

Five to 10 percent of people with high blood pressure have a type called secondary hypertension. Underlying it is a specific, and usually correctable, cause. If your hypertension came on very suddenly, developed early or late in life, or doesn't respond quickly to medication, your doctor may look for hidden causes. These include medical conditions such as thyroid dysfunction, obstructive sleep apnea, Cushing's syndrome, kidney failure, and high levels of aldosterone, a hormone that helps regulate fluid levels in the bloodstream. Your doctor may also check to see if you're taking any drugs or supplements that can raise blood pressure. These include oral contraceptives, pain-relieving nonsteroidal anti-inflammatories (like ibuprofen or naproxen), herbs (like ginseng or ma huang), steroids, decongestants, and diet pills.

---

pressure 6 points higher. However, experts say smoking over time is not a cause of high blood pressure. But by damaging artery walls, a tobacco habit accelerates the accumulation of heart-threatening plaque, boosting your risk for a heart attack or stroke to new heights if you also have high blood pressure. The fix: Quit! New research shows that former smokers can lower their heart attack risk to that of people who have never smoked.[23]

Body-Wide Damage: The Effects of High Blood Pressure

The force of blood under high pressure rips at the fragile inner lining of arteries throughout your body. This opens the door for a buildup of fatty plaque that threatens your heart and brain. The microscopic rips and tears also cause scarring. But the damage isn't limited to your cardiovascular system. By interfering with the blood supply to your organs, high blood pressure threatens your kidneys, eyes, brain, and, for men, sexual organs. The body chemistry changes behind high blood pressure also jeopardize bone health. Here's a more detailed look at the widespread effects of high blood pressure on your body.

Heart disease: Approximately 69 percent of people who have a first heart attack and 74 percent of people with congestive heart failure have high blood pressure.[24] Every 20-point increase in systolic BP or 10-point increase in diastolic BP doubles your risk for a fatal heart attack.[25] High blood pressure contributes to atherosclerosis (the buildup of plaque in your arteries) and, by stressing your heart, makes it grow thicker and stiffer. And researchers from the Montreal Heart Institute found that people with high blood pressure are less likely to notice mild chest pain, so they may miss the signs of a "silent" heart attack.[26]

Stroke: It only takes a tiny clot or microscopic rip in a blood vessel to trigger a stroke. These brain attacks destroy precious neurons by cutting off the supply of blood and oxygen. Each year, 795,000 Americans have a stroke; 129,000 die while tens of thousands are disabled. High blood pressure is the most potent risk factor for a stroke, raising the risk fourfold compared to people with normal blood pressure levels. Seventy-seven percent of people who have a first stroke have hypertension.[27] A 10-point increase in systolic

Is High Blood Pressure Keeping You Awake?

Obstructive sleep apnea (OSA), which occurs when tissue in your throat blocks breathing repeatedly through the night, can raise your blood pressure. But now, researchers suspect that high blood pressure may cause this sleep problem. Half of all people with OSA also have high blood pressure. Clearing up OSA via weight loss, surgery, or devices that keep airways open for better nighttime breathing can help control hypertension.[33] If you have high blood pressure and signs of OSA—loud nighttime snoring or daytime sleepiness—tell your doctor. And if you have OSA, stay on top of your blood pressure.

blood pressure can raise your risk for a fatal stroke by 15 to 28 percent.[28] Even prehypertension boosts risk 55 percent.[29]

Kidney problems: High blood pressure can damage the large arteries leading to your kidneys as well as hair-thin arteries that help filter waste from your bloodstream. Scarring of these tiny sieves can lead to kidney failure. Meanwhile, hypertension can also make blood vessels in your kidneys bulge, leading to a life-threatening rupture. Raised blood pressure is the second-leading cause of kidney failure. In a Spanish study of 5,551 people with hypertension or prehypertension, one in five had signs of kidney damage.[30]

Vision loss: At the back of your eyes, your retina works like a reverse movie screen, turning colors and images into signals sent to your brain. Hypertension can slowly steal your vision by damaging blood vessels in your retina. Ultimately, your eyesight may dim, you may experience double vision, or you may have headaches. This is hypertensive retinopathy, a problem for 2 to 14 percent of people over age 40.[31]

Dementia: When blood vessels within your brain tighten or become blocked by plaque, cells don't receive nourishment. This can lead to dementia. High blood pressure, it turns out, can also shrink some brain regions, leading to memory loss and fuzzy thinking up to a decade later, according to a recent study from Boston University.[32]

Erectile dysfunction (ED): Reduced bloodflow hampers a man's ability to achieve and sustain an erection. While hypertension isn't the only cause

(continued on page 28)

Success Story: *Tom Colbaugh*

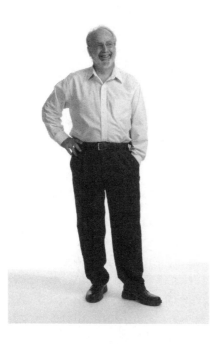

AGE: 59

HEIGHT: 5'11½"

BLOOD PRESSURE IMPROVEMENT:
Tom's systolic pressure fell 30 points and his diastolic pressure fell 17 points in 4 weeks.

POUNDS LOST: 14½

"This diet absolutely set me straight," says Tom. "I've had high blood pressure and type 2 diabetes for a long time. Before I started the plan, I was eating whatever I wanted. My blood pressure and my blood sugar were not under control. I was getting worried that I would have a heart attack or a stroke. The improvements have been amazing."

Tom's blood pressure fell from a dangerously high 193/82 to 163/65 in just 4 weeks. The dramatic improvement vastly reduced his risk for a heart attack or stroke, but his numbers were still high. Not for long, though. Tom continued following the plan. Four weeks later, he'd lost a total of 20 pounds and brought his blood pressure down to a definitely healthy 127/57. Working with his doctor, he's reduced his blood pressure and blood sugar medications, too.

"I saw my doctor right after the program ended, and based on my results, my drugs were reduced," he says. "I had been taking four or five pills twice a day for my blood pressure. Now I'm down to taking three pills once a day. My blood sugar levels are also lower, and my doctor reduced the doses of the medications I take for diabetes as well. He really liked my numbers."

After working as an organic livestock farmer for a decade, Tom changed careers while participating in the Lower Your Blood Pressure Naturally plan. "I became a table games dealer at a local casino," he says.

"I stuck with the plan because my wife supported me all the way, sharing the meals and exercising with me. She's lost 25 pounds on the plan."

The couple took a walk together almost every day. "I think that helped me a lot," Tom says. "I'm in pretty good shape—I'm a downhill ski instructor in the winter—but regular walks helped me reduce stress. So did yoga and a breathing exercise I do daily with a device called Resperate." (For more details about this device, see Chapter 15.)

The pair also adjusted the meal plan, swapping out foods like bananas and white potatoes that raise Tom's blood sugar. "Different foods affect people's blood sugar differently," he says. "I have to avoid these. I just eat more vegetables instead of having the bananas. I also decided to cut out caffeine because I realized, by checking with my blood pressure monitor and blood sugar meter, that it raises my blood pressure and my blood sugar."

He also realized that salt makes his blood pressure rise fast. "Cutting back on salt the first week let me drop several pounds and see a real improvement in my blood pressure," he says. "But I really noticed the effect of salt when I drank a margarita with a salted rim. My blood pressure jumped 20 points. So I keep my salt levels low now. I'll use a little on tomatoes or when I'm cooking chicken, but that's it."

The eating style that brought him so much success has become a new way of living. "I eat dinner at work. They provide a meal for us, and I make smart choices," he says. "I always have a green vegetable and a protein, like chicken or fish. I walk right past the pasta and sauce now. I want to make sure I'm getting lots of minerals and not so much sodium. I figure if I eat this way, I have a long life ahead of me."

of ED, it's a major factor. In one Israeli study of 1,412 men with ED, 38 percent had hypertension and another 25 percent had hypertension plus diabetes.[34] Sometimes erectile dysfunction is the first sign that something else is physically wrong, whether it be hypertension or cardiovascular disease.

Osteoporosis: If you have hypertension, your body may be getting rid of extra calcium in your urine as it tries to reduce levels of sodium in your bloodstream. Losing calcium may threaten bone health, boosting risk for a fracture.[35] In a 2013 study of 3,301 postmenopausal women, researchers from Italy's Gaetano Pini Institute found that 33 percent of participants with hypertension also had osteoporosis, compared to 23 percent without hypertension.[36]

CHAPTER 3

The Truth about Sodium

We wouldn't blame you for dumping extra salt on your french fries after hearing crazy, mixed-up news headlines like these: "Now Salt Is Safe to Eat," "No Benefit Seen in Sharp Limits on Salt in Diet," and even "Low-Sodium Diet Can Cause Problems."

But don't tip that saltshaker just yet!

The truth is, reducing your sodium intake the right way—as you will on the Lower Your Blood Pressure Naturally plan—is crucial for better BP. Don't let the widely misunderstood "salt wars" raging in parts of the scientific community and in the media keep you away from this essential, research-proven strategy. Our moderate sodium plan is based on the latest good science and is designed to make cutting back on salt easier, more effective, and more delicious than ever before.

Why Sodium Still Counts

Those news stories knocking low-salt diets got it wrong. New research underscores the importance of cutting out excess salt for everyone. Recent studies reveal four big reasons.

1. Too much sodium really does boost blood pressure. When Harvard Medical School scientists tracked sodium intake and blood pressure numbers of 8,208 people for 6 years, they concluded in 2012 that a high-salt diet is responsible for up to 40 percent of high blood pressure cases in America.[1] Problems start even before your numbers climb into the hypertensive range,

140/90 and above. In another recent study, sodium-packed eating increased risk for prehypertension—the stage before full-blown high blood pressure, with BP numbers between 120/80 and 139/89—by as much as 86 percent.[2]

It only takes a little excess sodium to nudge your numbers in the wrong direction. Increasing your daily intake by 1 gram—the amount in a scant half-teaspoon of salt or a small mug of canned chicken noodle soup—could boost your odds for high blood pressure by as much as 18 percent and for prehypertension by 5 percent, the researchers report. Bigger increases lead to bigger trouble. One 2013 study found that increasing salt intake by about a teaspoon a day could increase risk for a stroke by 23 percent and for heart disease by 17 percent.[3]

2. Reduced sodium intake tames elevated blood pressure. If high sodium increases risk, does reducing sodium help tame it? Recent, well-designed studies offer a definitive "yes." Three reports published in the *British Medical Journal* in 2013 analyzed more than 90 sodium/blood pressure studies and concluded that cutting back on salt reduces systolic blood pressure (the top number, an important indicator of heart health in people over age 50) by 4 points and drops diastolic blood pressure (the bottom number) by 2 points. That's not small. People who made these changes lowered their risk for heart attacks, strokes, and heart failure.[4] The more people cut back, the better their blood pressure numbers. Those who sliced their intake in half—from 5,580 milligrams to about 3,000 milligrams a day—reduced systolic and diastolic pressure by nearly 2 extra points.

That's significant. Every 5-point drop in systolic blood pressure reduces your risk for a stroke by 14 percent, heart disease by 9 percent, and an early death from any cause by 7 percent. Translation: You increase your chances for a longer, healthier life. That's what the citizens of Finland discovered. Researchers in that Scandinavian country report that when residents cut their salt intake 30 to 35 percent as part of a national health campaign, risk for fatal strokes and heart attacks fell by a dramatic 75 to 80 percent over 30 years.[5] As a result, Finns who cut back on salt lived an additional 6 to 7 years.

3. Keeping sodium in check matters for everyone. Some experts as well as spokespeople for the salt industry maintain that regulating sodium intake only matters for the estimated one in three people deemed salt-sensitive, meaning their bodies seem to retain more sodium and their blood pressure seems to react more strongly to it. It's true that in short-term studies, some people's blood pressure responds more dramatically to changes in salt intake. But thinking you've got a pass to indulge because you're *not* salt-sensitive is dangerous.

First, there's no test for salt sensitivity. We just don't know yet how to tell who's got the genes that may trigger a bigger reaction to a plate of salty nachos. Second, even if you're not genetically predisposed, you may be among the majority of Americans whose blood pressure is overreacting to sodium for lifestyle reasons. Studies show that BP levels are extra-sensitive to sodium if you are overweight (that's 70 percent of American adults), have a heart disease risk called metabolic syndrome (that's 34 percent of Americans),[6] or don't get enough pressure-controlling potassium and calcium in your diet (that's 98 percent of Americans). Third, studies of salt sensitivity only look at short-term drops in blood pressure when people cut back on salt for a few hours, days, or weeks. Longer-term studies show that keeping a lid on sodium has blood pressure benefits for almost everyone.

4. Reducing sodium can help your BP even if you take blood pressure medications. Is your BP still too high despite your (and your doctor's) efforts to control it with one, two, or even three medications? The missing ingredient in your treatment plan may be less sodium, says a recent study

---

Deciphering Sodium Claims

Wondering what those labels promising less sodium really deliver? Here's what the label claims mean.

- **"SODIUM FREE" OR "SALT FREE":** Provides less than 5 milligrams of sodium per serving
- **"UNSALTED" OR "NO SALT ADDED":** Contains no salt
- **"VERY LOW IN SODIUM":** Has 35 milligrams of sodium or less per serving
- **"LOW IN SODIUM" OR "CONTAINS A SMALL AMOUNT OF SODIUM":** Contains 140 milligrams of sodium or less per serving
- **"REDUCED SODIUM" OR "LESS SODIUM":** Has at least 25 percent less sodium than the traditional product

---

from Australia's Princess Alexandra Hospital. The study was small, yet hailed among cardiologists as "striking." Twelve people with resistant hypertension lowered their blood pressure in just a week when they cleaned up their diets by reducing sodium. They still needed medication, but side-stepped the prospect of more pills and increased doses. "In patients with resistant hypertension, a low-salt diet may be more effective than increasing the number of antihypertensive medications," the researchers concluded.[7]

How Low Should You Go?

The Lower Your Blood Pressure Naturally plan provides a moderate 2,300 milligrams of sodium a day. The plan is adjustable, allowing you to further reduce your intake if recommended by your doctor. Our realistic approach allows you to slash sodium to a level that helps control BP while enjoying fresh, flavorful meals, snacks, and desserts at home, and it gives you the flexibility to eat out and even grab fast, no-cook meals from the supermarket on busy days.

Ninety percent of us currently get far more sodium than the 2,300 milligrams a day recommended for most Americans by the Centers for Disease Control and Prevention.[8] Our average intake is a bloated 3,000 to 3,600 milligrams a day, according to national surveys from the US Department of Agriculture.[9] And 25 percent of us down far more than that. One in four women gets an average of 3,562 milligrams a day, and one in four men takes in 4,997 milligrams daily. One in 10 adults gets a whopping 4,690 to 6,470 milligrams of sodium daily.

Why does this plan call for 2,300 milligrams a day instead of going lower?

- **It works synergistically.** As you'll read later in this chapter and in the next one, combining a moderate sodium intake with other proven pressure-lowering strategies magnifies the benefits. Upping your consumption of calcium, magnesium, and potassium and losing pounds (and belly fat) as you cut back on sodium drives blood pressure down further than simply reducing sodium. Adding exercise and stress reduction lowers BP even more. Research shows that some of these approaches—like boosting your Power Mineral intake and getting exercise—can also keep your natural blood pressure regulation system from overreacting to the sodium you do eat. You may never have to go lower!

- **It's sustainable and delicious.** The benefits of maintaining a moderate salt diet are clear. Since most of us eat way too much sodium right now, we think 2,300 milligrams a day is a smart and powerful move in the right direction. Our test panelists discovered they never missed the excess salt. Cravings for it vanished, and high-sodium foods became decidedly unappealing. Panelists truly retrained their tastebuds to appreciate the flavors of foods naturally low in sodium and to savor seasonings or just a tiny sprinkle of salt. They never felt deprived.

Sodium Synergy

One of the most exciting discoveries in recent years about sodium and blood pressure actually concerns other minerals. It turns out that consuming more calcium, magnesium, and potassium while keeping your sodium in check magnifies the BP benefits.

Numbers tell the story. If you simply cut back on sodium, your blood pressure numbers could fall 2 to 8 points. Pretty good, and certainly enough to lower your risk for a heart attack or stroke. Go a step further by munching plenty of fresh, delicious foods loaded with BP-friendly minerals—exactly what you'll do on this plan—and you could subtract an additional 8 to 14 points.[10] Some of our test panelists got even more dramatic results as they

---

Salt or Sodium?

While we, and many experts, use the words *salt* and *sodium* interchangeably, they're not exactly the same thing. Table salt is sodium chloride, a mix of 40 percent sodium and 60 percent chloride.

- ¼ teaspoon salt = 581 milligrams sodium
- ½ teaspoon salt = 1,163 milligrams sodium
- ¾ teaspoon salt = 1,744 milligrams sodium
- 1 teaspoon salt = 2,325 milligrams sodium

---

enjoyed meals, snacks, and desserts built from Power Foods high in calcium, magnesium, and potassium (the nutrients we call Power Minerals).

Power Minerals work hard to promote healthier blood pressure at a cellular level. In fact, recent research shows that our bodies are designed to thrive on the proper balance of these three minerals in relation to sodium. (Read more in Chapter 4.) Yet most of us get too much sodium and way too little of the other three. You need 1,200 milligrams of calcium, 420 milligrams of magnesium, and 4,700 milligrams of potassium a day for maximum good health (and great BP), according to the US Department of Agriculture. Yet 98 percent of us don't get enough potassium, most of us don't eat enough foods with magnesium,[11] and the majority of women and men over age 50 shortchange themselves on dietary calcium, too.[12] Falling short, especially on potassium, actually enhances sodium's harmful effects, meaning even a little too much salt could send your blood pressure skyward.

Research shows that balancing the ratio of potassium to sodium in your diet gets the best results. The optimal ratio is 2:1, twice as much potassium as sodium or better. That's the ratio you'll feed your body on the Lower Your Blood Pressure Naturally plan. When that ratio is off-kilter, with more sodium and less potassium, risk for heart attacks, strokes, artery-clearing heart surgeries, and heart disease–related deaths rose in one 2009 study that tracked 3,000 people for 10 to 15 years. "Our study suggests that just lowering sodium, or just raising potassium, won't be nearly as effective for fighting hypertension or heart disease as doing both together," note the researchers from Harvard-affiliated Brigham and Women's Hospital in Boston.[13]

Bonus: Easier Weight Loss

Shedding excess weight is easier when you cut sodium. Health experts, including David A. Kessler, MD, former head of the US Food and Drug Administration, suspect that processed foods saturated with salt (along with sugar and fat) may trigger brain chemical changes that lead to cravings. That's on top of the extra calories you may be downing if you quench your salt-induced thirst with calorie-packed beverages.

Weight loss is a widely accepted lifestyle strategy for lowering blood pressure. But when you slash sodium at the same time, the effect is even bigger. According to a 2013 study from Massachusetts General Hospital, published in the journal *Hypertension,* people who used both strategies dropped their blood pressure further than those who used just one or the other.[14]

Losing weight, especially deep abdominal fat, can also help your body's BP-regulation system react in a healthier way to the salt you do eat. Tulane University researchers report that metabolic syndrome—a collection of heart disease and diabetes risks, including excess belly fat, low levels of "good" HDL cholesterol, high triglycerides, rising blood sugar, and rising blood pressure—triples the risk for salt sensitivity.[15] Research suggests that chronic, body-wide inflammation fueled by chemicals released from belly fat encourages sodium retention, which in turn can raise blood pressure. It may be no coincidence that half of all people with high blood pressure are overweight.[16]

This plan's efficient fat-blasting exercise plan also helps. Research shows that just 30 minutes of movement a day can reduce risk for salt-sensitive pressure changes by a whopping 38 percent.[17]

Inside the "Salt Wars"

If the evidence for keeping a lid on sodium is so convincing, why all the controversy? One reason is the gap between what consumers, the media, and heart researchers consider a low-sodium diet.

To consumers (including those in the news media), going low sodium generally means taking the saltshaker off the table and choosing more reduced- and low-sodium foods. But to the experts, a low-sodium diet is a specific, salt-restricted eating plan that slashes levels to just 1,500 milligrams a day. That's the level recommended currently by the American Heart Association for people with hypertension or at high risk for high blood pressure.

We'll be honest. Some people with hypertension do need to go that low to see results. And the Lower Your Blood Pressure Naturally plan can be adjusted to get you close to that number. But you may find that our "sodium synergy" approach gets you there without that drastic cut. That's the experience of several of our test panelists whose long-standing hypertension wasn't completely controlled with medications.

Since 2011, four major scientific reports have tried to assess the risks and benefits of extremely unsalty diets but ended up creating a bum rap for going low sodium. Critics say all of the reports were misunderstood by the media and also seriously flawed. None were gold-standard studies that tracked people who followed low-sodium diets. Instead, all analyzed older heart health studies that gathered limited data about participants' sodium intakes. Many did not consider that sicker people may have been more likely to try low-sodium eating, so poor health may have accounted for their poor outcomes. The results made low-sodium eating sound like a dud or even downright dangerous.[18] A 2011 British report analyzed seven studies involving more than 6,000 people and concluded that low-sodium eating didn't protect against fatal heart attacks.[19] A Danish analysis, also from 2011, looked at 167 studies and announced that low-salt eating did reduce blood pressure but might boost levels of some blood fats.[20] An international team of scientists, in another 2011 report, reviewed two studies involving nearly 29,000 people with heart risks and found that both high- and low-sodium diets appeared to raise risk for fatal heart attacks.[21]

Go Low, Go Natural

Five dramatic examples of how choosing natural foods—as you will on the Lower Your Blood Pressure Naturally plan—keeps sodium levels low.

NATURAL FOOD (1 SERVING)	SODIUM LEVEL	PROCESSED FOOD (1 SERVING)	SODIUM LEVEL
Apple	2 mg	Fast-food apple pie	400 mg
Fresh corn	1 mg	Canned corn	384 mg
Cucumber	2 mg	Dill pickle	928 mg
Potato	5 mg	Instant mashed potatoes	485 mg
Fresh tuna	50 mg	Fast-food fish sandwich	882 mg
Unsalted peanuts	8 mg	Dry-roasted, salted peanuts	986 mg
Tomato	14 mg	Ketchup (1 tablespoon)	154 mg

Then, in 2013, a new report from the Institute of Medicine (IOM) summed up what we know (and don't know) about sodium and cardiovascular health. This prestigious, government-appointed medical panel concluded that there just wasn't enough evidence to assess the benefits or harms of extremely low-sodium eating, in part because older studies were so seriously flawed. However, the IOM also concluded that eating lots of sodium does increase risk for heart and blood vessel problems.

What did the media say? "Eat Salt!" The headlines got it wrong again. The mistake even prompted IOM president Harvey V. Fineberg to write a letter to the US Department of Health and Human Services straightening out the confusion. Fineberg noted that "some press coverage misstated" the report's conclusions. He explained that reducing sodium was as important as ever. "The evidence linking sodium intake to health outcomes supports current efforts by the Centers for Disease Control and Prevention (CDC) and other authoritative bodies to reduce sodium intake in the US population below the current average adult intake of 3,400 mg per day," he wrote.[22]

Another health expert let off steam online. "The *Times* and some other media outlets undercut what should be the most important take-home message for consumers—consume less sodium," Michael F. Jacobson, executive director, Center for Science in the Public Interest, wrote on the group's Web site.[23] "Just gradually reducing our sodium intake to 2,300 milligrams a day, about a 40 percent reduction for most people, would yield enormous benefits. Doing so would save an estimated 280,000 to 500,000 lives, as well as about $90 billion in medical costs over the next decade," he added in a *Huffington Post* blog.[24]

In other words, it's time for a reality check about sodium. Since most of us eat way too much of it, worrying about the dubious ill effects of an extremely low-salt diet is beside the point. Reducing your intake to a moderate, sustainable, flavorful level for life is what counts.

Sodium in Your Body

Your body needs sodium to stay healthy. This mineral helps control blood pressure by playing an important role in maintaining the fluid balance in your bloodstream. It also aids the transmission of signals in your nervous system and helps muscles expand and contract. Without some sodium in your diet, you couldn't take a stroll in the park, heft a bag of groceries, grab a ringing cell phone from your purse, or receive important messages delivered by your nerves to your brain, like "I'm full; stop eating," "Ouch, that wasp just stung my hand," or "Oh, that was a lovely kiss!"

Sodium is so crucial for survival in nature that animals risk their lives to visit salt licks. And for prehistoric humans, who ate a naturally low-sodium diet, a taste for salt may have ensured survival.

But today, salt is no longer scarce. Most of us never have to worry about getting too little. Our bodies need just 200 to 500 milligrams of sodium a day (less than ¼ teaspoon salt) for healthy functioning, yet we get far more.

Your kidneys help maintain ideal sodium levels by retaining this mineral if blood levels drop too low and by getting rid of excess when levels rise too high. But your body also balances fluid and sodium levels by triggering a "thirsty" signal when sodium levels rise, prompting you to drink more liquids and add more water to the system. And the hormone vasopressin is released by your pituitary gland, telling your kidneys to hold on to more urine. As a result, the amount of water in your bloodstream increases to better balance sodium levels.

Trouble happens when sodium levels stay too high for too long. The amount of water in your bloodstream stays high. And, like rainwater swelling a mountain stream after a storm, the force of the blood in your circulatory system increases. Your heart works harder.[25] And your blood pressure rises.[26]

But science has also found that extra salt boosts BP by damaging blood vessels. In a 2012 study, Harvard Medical School researchers tracked the sodium intakes of 5,556 men and women from the Netherlands for 6 years. People who consumed the most sodium had more uric acid and albumin in their urine, markers of blood vessel damage. Compared to those who got less than 2,200 milligrams of sodium a day, those with high-salt diets were 21 percent more likely to develop high blood pressure. Risk was 32 to 86 percent higher for those who also had high uric acid or albumin levels.[27]

Where's the Salt?

Even if you're careful with your saltshaker, you may be getting way more than you think. Just 5 to 6 percent of sodium is sprinkled on food at the table; another 5 to 6 percent is added in cooking, and a smidge is found naturally in edibles like vegetables, dairy products, and seafood. More than 75 percent of the sodium we eat is hidden in packaged, processed, and restaurant foods.[28] And there's more there than you may think. In one national survey, restaurant patrons underestimated the sodium in popular entrées by as much as 90 percent.[29] Even seemingly healthy fare—like whole grain bread, tomato sauce, and low-fat lunchmeats—can pack a salty wallop.

A 2012 report from the CDC pinpointed the worst culprits (see "Top 10 Sodium Sources in the American Diet," below). Forty-four percent of the sodium Americans consume comes from just 10 food categories: bread, cold cuts and cured meats, pizza, poultry, soups, sandwiches, cheese, pasta mixed dishes, meat mixed dishes, and savory snacks.[30] The researchers note that trimming the sodium in just these foods by 25 percent could prevent 28,000 deaths and save $7 billion in health care costs per year.

How salty are the top 10? With 150 milligrams of sodium or more in a small handful, potato chips and pretzels are no surprise. Bread and rolls don't seem particularly salty, but we eat so much of them that the sodium they do contain adds up. A single slice of bread may contain 230 milligrams,

Top 10 Sodium Sources in the American Diet

A recent Centers for Disease Control and Prevention survey found that these foods contain 44 percent of the sodium we eat.

1. Bread and rolls, 7.4%
2. Cold cuts and cured meats, 5.1%
3. Pizza, 4.9%
4. Fresh and processed poultry, 4.5%
5. Soups, 4.3%
6. Sandwiches (like cheeseburgers), 4%
7. Cheese, 3.8%
8. Pasta mixed dishes (like spaghetti with meat sauce), 3.3%
9. Meat mixed dishes (like meat loaf with tomato sauce), 3.2%
10. Savory snacks (including chips, pretzels, popcorn, and puffs), 3.1%

10 percent of your daily total on a moderate-sodium eating plan. Layer on a serving of deli turkey and you'll add about 900 milligrams. Meanwhile, a slice of pepperoni pizza can contain more than 950 milligrams, and $\frac{1}{2}$ cup of pasta sauce can tack on 470 milligrams or more. An ounce of cheese can deliver anywhere from 54 milligrams for Swiss to 263 milligrams for processed American and 395 milligrams for blue cheese. Just $\frac{1}{2}$ cup of canned chicken noodle soup packs 890 milligrams. And while untreated chicken is very low in sodium (about 70 milligrams per serving), an uncooked chicken breast from the supermarket could contain salty broth to enhance flavor, raising the sodium level to a shocking 440 milligrams. Other surprising sources include cottage cheese (up to 900 milligrams per cup), bottled salad dressing (up to 300 milligrams in 2 tablespoons), canned vegetables (up to 800 milligrams in 1 cup of green beans), canned beans (700 milligrams), ready-to-eat cereal (350 milligrams or more per cup), and soy sauce (533 milligrams in 1 tablespoon).

Many food makers are working to slice back the salt in processed foods through the National Salt Reduction Initiative. The goal: Cut sodium levels by an average of 25 percent by 2014. But we're not there yet. Recent research by the Center for Science in the Public Interest found that sodium levels fell an average of 3.5 percent between 2005 and 2011 in 402 analyzed foods. But a closer look showed that sodium increased in one in four products tested, by as much as 30 percent.[31] At the same time, levels in restaurant meals increased by 2.6 percent. Canadian researchers recently found that the average restaurant meal contains 2,269 milligrams of sodium—a day's worth.[32] Even hospital food contains twice as much salt as it should, University of Toronto researchers announced in 2012.[33]

Why all the salt? This mineral works as a flavor enhancer that also extends shelf life, adds tenderness to cured meats (by plumping up the proteins with extra water), improves the color of hot dogs, and contributes to the appealing golden brown hue of the crusts on baked goods. It appears on ingredient labels in many chemical guises for even more uses. Sodium bicarbonate (baking soda) makes baked goods rise. Sodium caseinate is a binder used in nondairy creamers, nondairy toppings, and desserts. Sodium erythorbate prevents color and flavor changes. Sodium propionate inhibits mold growth in puddings, jams, cheese, and gelatins. Sodium lactate stops the growth of bacteria in cured meats.

Reset Your Tastebuds

Test panelists—even those who had absolutely loved salty foods—were pleased and surprised to discover that they lost their taste for overly salty foods after a week or two on the Lower Your Blood Pressure Naturally plan. Panelist Chris Colbaugh found he could barely eat a once-favorite red meat dish. Penny Boos felt shocked at the levels of salt in foods eaten away from home.

Research shows that as you eat less salt, your tastebuds recover their natural appreciation for a wide range of flavors. In one study from Philadelphia's Monell Chemical Senses Center, people rated the saltiness of crackers and soup as less pleasant after following a low-sodium diet for a few weeks.[34] After a few months, foods they'd enjoyed before the start of the study were deemed "too salty."

The good news is, you don't have to completely eliminate salt to reset your tastebuds. Our plan retains a small amount to enhance the flavors of foods. And it does so in the most effective way possible: by sprinkling on a few grains just before serving. A little "surface sodium" boosts flavor more than sodium added during cooking. Our recipes call for kosher salt or coarse sea salt. By weight, these contain the exact same amount of sodium as table salt. But the large flakes mean that you get less salt by volume when you measure it out. (There's more space between the grains.) You'll save about 10 milligrams of sodium per 1/8 teaspoon salt this way.

A Better Sodium Plan

On the Lower Your Blood Pressure Naturally eating plan, you'll feast on meals, snacks, and desserts naturally low in sodium and high in pressure-controlling calcium, magnesium, and potassium. You'll enjoy ingredients like sweet peaches and bananas, satisfying bulgur and quinoa, hearty pork tenderloin and tilapia, and luscious avocados.

And you'll discover delicious recipes so full of flavor, you won't notice that you've reduced your salt intake. How about Corn Tortilla Pizzas

Does Anyone Need More Sodium?

It's relatively rare, but in a condition called hyponatremia, sodium levels in the blood fall dangerously low. It may be triggered by conditions like heart or kidney failure or by not drinking fluids with electrolytes (sodium and other minerals) after endurance exercise in the heat. Water pills (diuretics) and some antidepressants and pain pills that prompt you to urinate or perspire more than usual can also deplete sodium. So can prolonged illnesses with diarrhea and vomiting.

Hyponatremia can cause brain swelling. Symptoms include confusion, headaches, restlessness, fatigue, muscle spasms, nausea and vomiting, and even seizures and unconsciousness. Severe, sudden hyponatremia may be treated with intravenous sodium and medications.

(page 120) for dinner? Chopped Chicken Salad (page 118) for lunch? Cheesy Potato Hash Topped with an Egg (page 111) for breakfast? Peanut Butter–Banana Frozen Yogurt (page 129) or Double-Dark Hot Chocolate (page 128) for dessert? It's all waiting for you.

CHAPTER 4

Power Minerals: The Key to Healthy Blood Pressure

How about starting your day with a Creamy Banana Smoothie (page 89) that gets a flavor boost from a surprising, mineral-packed "secret" ingredient, sweet potato? Or serving a flavorful pork tenderloin for Sunday dinner, paired with broccoli (drizzled with olive oil and lemon juice) and a delicious whole grain? Or sitting down to a filling Veggie and Cheddar Frittata (page 113) or Open-Faced Tuna Melt (page 117) for lunch?

You'll savor these fabulous foods and many more in your first week on the Lower Your Blood Pressure Naturally eating plan. Amazingly, every breakfast, lunch, and dinner recipe is made with just 13 specially chosen Power Foods that deliver the latest nutritional strategy for optimal blood pressure lowering: the synergy created by slashing sodium and increasing levels of the Power Minerals calcium, magnesium, and potassium.

As you learned in Chapter 3, it's not enough to just lower sodium. High blood pressure really responds when you restore the natural mineral balance your body needs for healthy BP regulation. Off-kilter levels are all too common in America, thanks to the overly salty, low-mineral diets most of us consume. A better plan? The one in this book. Based on cutting-edge research, it delivers the perfect mineral ratio: 2,300 milligrams of sodium along with 4,700 milligrams of potassium, 1,200 milligrams of calcium, and 420 milligrams of magnesium.

Here's why Power Minerals—and our Power Foods—promote healthy blood pressure.

Potassium: Striking a Powerful Balance with Sodium

Once upon a time, blood pressure experts thought that simply reducing sodium was the key to a great blood pressure–lowering diet. Now medical science understands that striking a healthy balance between sodium and potassium makes all the difference. The ideal ratio is 2:1, twice as much potassium as sodium. That's the balance you'll enjoy on the Lower Your Blood Pressure Naturally plan, as you can see from the numbers we gave you above.

More than 99 percent of Americans miss the mark though, report University of Washington researchers who reviewed the diets of 12,038 people for a 2012 study.[1] We overdo sodium, which abounds in packaged, processed, and restaurant foods, getting an average of 3,400 milligrams per day. And we fall short on potassium because we skimp on produce, low-fat dairy, beans, and other natural foods rich in this mineral, getting an average of just 2,640 milligrams a day, according to the US Department of Agriculture.[2]

In 2009, the consequences of this imbalanced eating came into sharp focus when Harvard Medical School researchers[3] reviewed the mineral intakes and health histories of 2,275 people. They found that striking a healthy balance cut risk for strokes, heart attacks, and heart blockages nearly in half. In 2011, a larger study confirmed the discovery. Researchers from the Centers for Disease Control and Prevention who reviewed 15 years of health records for 12,267 people found that those who got the most sodium and the least potassium doubled their odds for fatal heart disease.[4] People with the lowest rates of heart disease didn't just eat less salt or get more potassium; they did both. Simply cutting back on sodium or bumping up potassium alone wasn't nearly as protective.

That's synergy. It works because these two minerals work together in your body to perform important functions. Your body needs twice as much potassium as sodium to keep an important, energy-generating system in your cells functioning properly. It's called the sodium-potassium pump. If you're low on potassium, this pump produces by-products that can induce arteries to tighten up.[5, 6] Excess dietary sodium also boosts blood pressure by trapping extra water in your blood. Your kidneys normally dump extra sodium into your urine for excretion, but potassium goes with it; if levels of this mineral are low, your body holds on to excess sodium in order to keep more potassium on board. And while potassium helps arteries stay flexible by activating the release of a relaxing compound called nitric oxide in artery walls, sodium has the opposite effect: It blocks nitric oxide and makes artery walls stiff.[7]

Potassium on the Lower Your Blood Pressure Naturally Plan

You'll feast on delicious, unprocessed foods rich in potassium and naturally low in sodium, including peaches, kiwifruit, white beans, yogurt, sweet potatoes, and avocados. How about Peaches and Cream Hot Quinoa Cereal (page 87), with 1,050 milligrams of potassium and 167.7 milligrams of sodium; hearty Sweet Potato Hash (page 90), 1,426 milligrams of potassium and 343.5 milligrams of sodium; or Peanut Butter–Banana Frozen Yogurt (page 129), 517 milligrams of potassium and 129 milligrams of sodium?

Calcium: "Zen" for Your Arteries

Calcium's not just good for your bones. While 99 percent of your body's stockpile of this mineral is stored in your skeleton and teeth, the remaining 1 percent circulates in your bloodstream and moves in and out of your cells on an important mission. Calcium helps blood vessels contract and expand; it also aids the transmission of signals in nerves and cells. These tasks are so important that if blood levels of calcium are low, your body will rob calcium from your bones to make sure they happen.

When calcium intake is low, artery walls can tighten. Calcium also helps your body maintain a healthier sodium balance; low levels of calcium hamstring efforts to off-load this blood pressure–boosting mineral.[8]

But don't just pop a pill. Evidence is mounting that getting your calcium from food, as you will on this plan, rather than from a supplement is best for blood pressure control and a healthy heart. One reason: Dairy products deliver more than calcium. They also contain whey and casein, proteins that put the brakes on angiotensin converting enzyme, a compound that helps regulate blood pressure by tightening arteries and encouraging your kidneys to hold on to sodium.[9]

A University of South Carolina review of the health histories of 17,030 Americans found that those who got more calcium from food had lower increases in systolic blood pressure, an indicator of artery health, as they aged.[10] In contrast, relying on supplements might cause trouble.[11] In a massive National Institutes of Health study that followed 388,229 women and men for 15 years, researchers found that men who took 1,000 milligrams or more of supplemental calcium daily had a 20 percent higher risk for fatal heart disease.[12] However, calcium from food didn't raise risk. A Finnish study found similar risks for women.[13]

But don't conclude that simply skipping calcium is better. For one thing, you'll miss out on a crucial building block for strong bones. And research also suggests that getting too little of this mineral may raise heart risks.[14, 15]

Best calcium intake? You'll protect bones and reap blood pressure benefits with 1,200 milligrams a day, the amount recommended by the Institute of Medicine for people over age 50.[16] It's the same amount you'll enjoy on this plan. You may be surprised to discover that you're skimping on calcium-rich foods: One government survey found that most women as well as men over age 50 don't get enough.[17]

When combined with low-sodium, potassium-packed eating, calcium's blood pressure punch is bigger. Researchers suspect that even small shortfalls of calcium and potassium can create imbalances that tighten muscle cells in artery walls.[18] And in a landmark study of a mineral-rich food fix for high blood pressure, called Dietary Approaches to Stop Hypertension, people who ate foods rich in both calcium and potassium (along with magnesium) saw bigger BP drops than those who skipped calcium-rich dairy products.[19] At the end of the study, 70 percent of volunteers on the combination diet had lowered their blood pressure to healthy levels, compared to just 45 percent who ate loads of produce but didn't add daily calcium-rich dairy.[20]

Calcium on the Lower Your Blood Pressure Naturally Plan

You'll enjoy just-right levels of daily calcium from yogurt and fat-free milk (or a dairy alternative such as soy milk) as well as from surprising plant sources, including broccoli, kale, quinoa, and white beans. How about a cup of Double-Dark Hot Chocolate (page 128), with 330 milligrams of calcium;

a Peach-Almond Ice Cream Cup (page 127), 150 milligrams of calcium; or Kale Salad with Roasted Peaches, Spiced Yogurt-Avocado Dressing, and Tilapia (page 93), 357 milligrams of calcium?

Magnesium: Quiet yet Mighty

The third member of our Power Mineral trio, magnesium, is emerging as an important player in heart health and better blood pressure. It helps potassium and calcium pass through cell walls to do their work.[21] This mineral also helps nitric oxide relax artery walls.[22] In 2013, Dutch researchers published two studies showing that low magnesium levels boost risk for heart attacks by 60 percent[23] and that high levels seem to lower risk for high blood pressure.[24]

In two big Harvard School of Public Health studies of 70,000 doctors and nurses, those with the highest magnesium intakes had healthier diastolic and systolic blood pressure numbers.[25] A University of Minnesota study of nearly 8,000 people found that risk for hypertension was 70 percent lower in women with the highest blood levels of magnesium and 18 percent lower in men.[26]

On this plan, you'll get 420 milligrams of magnesium a day from food, enough to satisfy women's and men's needs for optimal health. Up to 45 percent of us currently shortchange ourselves of this important mineral.[27] If you take blood pressure drugs, you should know that some diuretics (water pills) can also cause magnesium deficiencies.[28] Couldn't you just take a pill to make up the difference? Nope. Experts say the magnesium in food works better, in part because you get other pressure-pampering minerals at the same time.[29] Synergy at work yet again.

Magnesium on the Lower Your Blood Pressure Naturally Plan

You'll get the magnesium you need from kale, quinoa, sweet potatoes, pork, white beans, and other delicious edibles rich in this mineral. How about Tilapia with Kiwi-Avocado Salsa, Roasted Broccoli, and Quinoa (page 99), with 131 milligrams of magnesium; a Creamy Banana Smoothie (page 89), 93.8 milligrams of magnesium; or an Open-Faced Avocado-Mozzarella Egg Sandwich (page 108), 87.8 milligrams of magnesium?

Meet Our 13 Amazing Power Foods

The meals and smoothies you'll enjoy during the first week of this eating plan are all built with 13 delicious and versatile Power Foods. Eating plan developers Stephanie Clarke and Willow Jarosh, both registered dietitians with a flair for creating tastebud-pleasing, healthy recipes the whole family will love, chose these particular foods after reviewing the nutritional profiles of hundreds of possibilities.

We presented the two of them with a huge challenge: Create a palate of proteins, starches, vegetables, fruits, and good fats that met our stringent nutritional criteria. Each Power Food had to:

- Be naturally low in sodium
- Provide a significant percentage of the daily requirement for at least two of the three Power Minerals
- Deliver plenty of satisfying fiber, lean protein, or healthy fats along with other vitamins and minerals necessary for good health
- Be tasty, budget friendly, simple to find in any supermarket, easy to prepare, and versatile enough to work in a wide variety of breakfast, lunch, and dinner combinations
- Be naturally low in calories for weight loss

Impossible? Not for Stephanie and Willow. Our test panelists were delighted with these 13 amazing foods. You will be, too.

Proteins

White beans

Power Mineral profile: One cup of white beans provides 13 percent of the calcium, 30 percent of the magnesium, and 24 percent of the potassium you need every day.

Good to know: You'll use this comfort food in side dishes, a soup, and entrées, like Garlicky Kale and White Beans with Tilapia (page 95) and Pork and Veggie Taco Salad Slaw (page 97). The mild flavor of white beans is enhanced by our signature spice blends and garlic (if you desire). As a meatless source of protein, it's a great choice for vegetarians. Choose no-salt-added or well-rinsed low-sodium canned white beans, or cook dried beans overnight in a slow cooker.

Pork tenderloin

Power Mineral profile: Three ounces of pork tenderloin provide 6 percent of the magnesium and 15 percent of the potassium you need every day.

Good to know: Meat lovers, rejoice! This lean cut provides plenty of meaty flavor and satisfaction without the overload of saturated fat found in fattier types of beef and pork. You'll use it for Dukkah-Spiced Pork Tenderloin with Broccoli and Quinoa (page 96), a terrific family dinner; Red Bell Pepper Stuffed with Pork and Quinoa (page 100); and more. Cook larger tenderloins (or do several on the grill or in the oven) and store leftovers in the refrigerator or freezer for fast weeknight meals.

Fat-free plain yogurt

Power Mineral profile: One cup of fat-free plain yogurt provides 49 percent of the calcium, 12 percent of the magnesium, and 18 percent of the potassium you need every day.

Good to know: Cool and creamy, yogurt is a star ingredient in mineral-rich breakfasts like the Creamy Banana Smoothie (page 89), in sauces and salad dressings, and even in entrées like Twice-Baked Spiced Sweet Potato with Roasted Broccoli and Tilapia (page 91). We chose regular yogurt in Phase 1 instead of Greek varieties; most brands are a bit higher in calcium.

Tilapia

Power Mineral profile: Four ounces of tilapia provides 8 percent of the magnesium and 8 percent of the potassium you need every day.

Good to know: This mild white fish is available year-round in supermarkets and fish stores, fresh or as frozen fillets. You'll roast it, bake it, and sauté it, flavored with a variety of seasonings and even topped with mineral-rich kiwi-avocado salsa. Tilapia is extremely low in environmental toxins like mercury and PCBs (polychlorinated biphenyls), and it is considered a sustainable, environmentally friendly choice. Most US-raised tilapia is grown in closed-system fish farms on plant-based diets, an approach that doesn't threaten stocks of wild fish, according to the nonprofit Food & Water Watch.

Fruits

Kiwifruit

Power Mineral profile: One kiwifruit provides 2 percent of the calcium, 7 percent of the magnesium, and 9 percent of the potassium you need every day.

Good to know: Kiwifruit is available year-round in supermarkets, hailing from California orchards November through May and from New Zealand June through October. (Kiwifruit was named after New Zealand's native kiwi bird, whose brown, fuzzy coat resembles the skin of this fruit.) The sweet flavor might remind you of strawberries, bananas, or a ripe melon. Creamy and juicy, it is featured in our Green Machine Smoothie (page 88) and the Kiwi-Peach Yogurt Parfait (page 88), and it is paired with avocado as a salsa to top tilapia. Ripe kiwis can be stored in the fridge or on your counter. They contain more vitamin C than a same-size serving of orange slices.

Peaches and nectarines

Power Mineral profile: One medium peach or nectarine provides 1 percent of the calcium, 3 percent of the magnesium, and 8 percent of the potassium you need every day.

Good to know: So sweet, so juicy, and so versatile, peaches (or nectarines) made our Peaches and Cream Hot Quinoa Cereal (page 87) a hands-down favorite among test panelists. And we found a sophisticated new way to use this fruit: roasted, to bring out all that summer flavor in our Kale Salad with Roasted Peaches, Spiced Yogurt-Avocado Dressing, and Tilapia (page 93). Frozen unsweetened peach slices are a great alternative to fresh peaches and nectarines on the plan. Just defrost ahead of time or, for smoothies in Phase 2, simply toss in the blender.

Bananas

Power Mineral profile: One medium banana provides 1 percent of the calcium, 8 percent of the magnesium, and 12 percent of the potassium you need every day.

Good to know: High in potassium and magnesium, bananas are a mainstay of several Phase 1 smoothies. They lend a luxuriously creamy, sweet quality to blended drinks. No need to toss soft bananas when the skin turns brown. Peel, bag, and freeze for use in smoothies.

Vegetables

Kale

Power Mineral profile: One cup of kale, raw or cooked, provides 9 percent of the calcium, 6 percent of the magnesium, and 9 percent of the potassium you need every day.

Good to know: Drink your greens! The ruffled leaves of this superhealthy cruciferous vegetable are a major ingredient in our Phase 1 Green Machine Smoothie (page 88). This breakfast drink gets its sweetness from banana and kiwi and its creamy quality from yogurt and a little avocado. You'll find kale in our Phase 1 salads, in side dishes, and paired with white beans in soup. You'll also discover an interesting kale and avocado salad (page 101) that uses a new salad prep technique for extra softness and flavor: massaging greens with oil. While most recipes call for large amounts of salt to do this, our version uses a tiny, healthy ⅛ teaspoon of kosher salt to bring out kale's taste without a sodium overload.

Low in calories, kale is widely considered a superfood because it contains a big dose of cell-protecting antioxidants as well as alpha-linolenic acid, a plant-based good fat that cools inflammation. Thin, delicate baby kale leaves are a great alternative for salads.

Red bell pepper

Power Mineral profile: One cup of raw red bell pepper provides 1 percent of the calcium, 4 percent of the magnesium, and 9 percent of the potassium you need every day.

Good to know: Juicy and crunchy, red bell pepper is fun to eat raw. When cooked, it complements the flavors of other hearty eating plan ingredients like pork, broccoli, bulgur, and kale. Red bell pepper is the basis for our Red Bell Pepper Stuffed with Pork and Quinoa (page 100), and it lends extra appeal to our Massaged Kale Avocado Salad (page 101). Red bell peppers keep in the refrigerator for up to 10 days. Store wrapped in a slightly damp paper towel so they don't dry out. You can freeze extras to use later in cooked dishes.

Broccoli

Power Mineral profile: One cup of cooked broccoli provides 6 percent of the calcium, 8 percent of the magnesium, and 14 percent of the potassium you need every day.

Good to know: This cruciferous veggie is a famous source of cancer-fighting phytonutrients called glucosinolates, but don't overlook broccoli's heart-smart supply of all three pressure-soothing Power Minerals. We've tucked broccoli into plenty of Phase 1 meals, seasoned with garlic, roasted as a side dish, swirled in a stir-fry, or left raw and finely chopped in the Pork and Veggie Taco Salad Slaw (page 97). Fresh broccoli works best in the eating plan recipes, but you can substitute frozen in many cooked entrées and side dishes.

Food Starches

Sweet potato

Power Mineral profile: One medium sweet potato with the skin provides 4 percent of the calcium, 8 percent of the magnesium (7 percent without the skin), and 15 percent of the potassium (10 percent without the skin) you need every day.

Good to know: So sweet it could be a dessert, sweet potato is the secret ingredient in our Phase 1 Creamy Banana Smoothie (page 89). You'll also welcome this treat at lunch and dinner in dishes like Twice-Baked Spiced Sweet Potato with Roasted Broccoli and Tilapia (page 91) and meatless White Bean–Sweet Potato Patties over Kale Topped with Yogurt Sauce (page 94). Willow and Stephanie recommend baking several sweet potatoes at the start of Week 1 so you'll have a ready supply for quick smoothies and other recipes.

Quinoa

Power Mineral profile: A half-cup of cooked quinoa provides 1.5 percent of the calcium, 15 percent of the magnesium, and 4.5 percent of the potassium you need every day.

Good to know: There's a reason the United Nations declared 2013 the International Year of Quinoa. This high-protein whole grain has a mild yet nutty flavor, contains a variety of health-protecting phytonutrients along with an impressive amount of magnesium, and cooks in less than half the time it takes to make brown rice. In Phase 1, you'll enjoy quinoa in Peaches and Cream Hot Quinoa Cereal (page 87), Pork Stir-Fry with Quinoa (page 92), and Red Bell Pepper Stuffed with Pork and Quinoa (page 100).

Quinoa is gluten free, making it a great option if you're gluten intolerant or have celiac disease. The most widely available quinoa is a golden beige color, but red and black varieties are also available and worth a try.

Good Fat

Avocado
Power Mineral profile: One-half of an avocado provides 1 percent of the calcium, 5 percent of the magnesium, and 10 percent of the potassium you need every day.

Good to know: Luscious avocado is your go-to good fat for Phase 1 of this plan. You'll discover new ways to enjoy it, such as in smoothies, mixed with yogurt, in salsas and dressings, and in salads. In addition to pressure-soothing minerals and heart-healthy monounsaturated fats, avocados contain health-promoting carotenoids. Peel carefully; the dark green flesh just under an avocado's brittle skin contains large amounts of these disease-fighting compounds.

Success Story: *Bryon Boos*

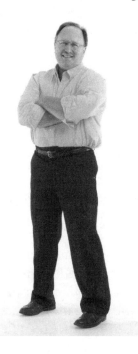

AGE: 54

HEIGHT: 5'8"

BLOOD PRESSURE IMPROVEMENT:
Bryon's systolic pressure fell 9 points
and his diastolic pressure fell 3 points in
4 weeks.

POUNDS LOST: 11

Bryon Boos isn't just busy by day.
Between his job managing a factory and
his avocation making wine, he's busy
around the clock. "When my doctor
wanted to put me on medicine for my
blood pressure, I knew it could be hard
to get out of that cycle—you're stressed
and don't have time to eat well, so you
end up taking more medicine," he says.
"When my wife told me about the plan,
I wanted to do it for myself and for her."

Penny Boos, Bryon's wife, was making healthy changes for herself in
the aftermath of a heart attack. "I wanted to support Penny," he says. "In
fact, that was my first motivation. We did the plan together. We totally
changed the way we eat and got great results."

Bryon's blood pressure fell from 131/77 to a healthier 122/74 in 4 weeks.
In addition to dropping 11 pounds, his waist size shrank 5¼ inches—a sign
that he was losing the abdominal fat that's an especially potent driver of
high blood pressure. "I wake up in the morning feeling better," he says.
"When you lose inches you feel better about yourself, and when you lose
weight you feel more confident."

Desalting their diets wasn't easy at first, he admits. "Eating foods with
less sodium takes some getting used to, but as we continued, our palates
really changed," he says. "If you know it's the healthy thing to do, it's a sac-
rifice you make. After a few weeks, we were used to it. And when we did
eat out, we really noticed how salty restaurant food is. Now we appreciate

the natural flavors in foods. It's a huge change. And since the plan is low in sugar, we've also become aware of how much sugar is added to restaurant food."

Favorite meals that the couple still makes at home include the Cheesy Potato Hash Topped with an Egg (page 111), the Orange-Carrot Creamsicle Smoothie (page 125), and the Tropical Greens Smoothie (page 124). "We went off the plan for a few weeks once it ended, but we've just recommitted to it," he says. "We want to maintain our progress."

Bryon admits that his busy schedule didn't leave time for all the components of the plan. "I didn't exercise or meditate," he says. "My reading might have been even better if I did. And we had a glass of wine once in a while. But I started checking my blood pressure more often. I think that's something everyone should just do at a certain point in life. Otherwise, how will you know what's happening?"

So what accounted for his success? "It was the diet," he says. "You're eliminating salt and sugar and getting the right minerals. That mix is key. It's really changed the way we prepare our food. We're making more conscious choices now when we shop and when we cook—even when we make foods that aren't in the plan. We got a salt-free seasoning mix last week to use on grilled chicken. It has white pepper in it and tastes wonderful, even though it makes me sneeze when I sprinkle it on! We've changed our habits for the better."

CHAPTER 5

Weight Loss, Exercise, Serenity, and More: The Magic of Synergy

Our test panelists are the proof: Combining the eight proven, drug-free strategies for taming blood pressure multiplies the benefits. That's the magic of synergy. While medical science has yet to study the full effect of this plan's unique and powerful approach, a growing stack of research shows that combining even a few of the elements in this plan turbocharges your BP payback. Just imagine what will happen when you incorporate all eight healthy changes into your life!

Here's what science has to say about the power of synergy for lowering blood pressure.

- **One healthy change = good.** In a Tulane University study of 975 people with high blood pressure, 36 to 40 percent of volunteers who reduced sodium or lost weight got their numbers out of the hypertension range.[1]

- **Two healthy changes = better.** In that same study, 53 percent of volunteers who slimmed down and dumped the salt from their diets improved blood pressure significantly.[2] Other research shows that while slashing sodium can lower BP 2 to 8 points, boosting calcium, magnesium, and potassium (the Power Minerals featured in this plan) at the same time can lower it an additional 8 to 14 points.[3]

- **Four healthy changes = wow!** In a multicenter study of 810 people with hypertension or prehypertension, those who made four lifestyle changes—eating more Power Minerals, getting regular exercise, losing weight, and slashing sodium—were the clear winners. Seventy-seven percent of participants with hypertension got their numbers out of the high blood pressure range, compared to 66 percent who lost weight, exercised, and cut sodium but didn't boost mineral intake.[4] Deploying all four strategies helped 48 percent of those with prehypertension get their numbers down into the healthy range, compared to 40 percent who didn't add more mineral-rich foods to their diets.

You've already learned about two of our eight approaches—reducing sodium to moderate levels (in Chapter 3) and hitting your daily Power Mineral quota with foods rich in calcium, magnesium, and potassium (in Chapter 4). Here's the lowdown on the other six strategies that are the building blocks of the Lower Your Blood Pressure Naturally plan.

Strategy: Weight Loss

Our healthy eating plan and time-saving exercise routine are designed to help you reach two goals: healthier blood pressure and a healthier body weight. The strategy works. Test panelists lost up to 14.4 pounds. They also trimmed inches from their thighs and hips and up to $5\frac{1}{4}$ inches from their waistlines. They're fitting into their skinny jeans, and they knocked back a potent blood pressure foe: body fat.

The connection between fat and hypertension is dramatic. A whopping 60 to 70 percent of high numbers are the direct result of extra pounds, notes a 2010 report in the *American Journal of Hypertension*.[5] And carrying extra weight boosts your odds for high blood pressure as much as sixfold![6, 7] In fact, tipping the bathroom scale by just 10 extra pounds can raise your pressure 4 points, enough to require hypertension medication and increase your risk for a heart attack or stroke. It's a common concern: 60 percent of women and men with high blood pressure are at least 20 percent overweight.[8] And carrying those pounds around your middle is dangerous. In a University of Michigan study of more than 24,000 people, a large waistline increased high blood pressure risk by about 50 percent.[9]

Losing extra pounds is a powerful solution. In one large study that tracked the weight and health histories of 36,075 women for up to 50 years, Vanderbilt University researchers found that those who had lost weight reduced their risk for prehypertension by 24 to 54 percent.[10] Simply losing weight, even if you don't take other healthy steps, helps. Experts estimate that every 2.2 pounds you lose reduces BP numbers up to 3 points.[11, 12] Losing 5 to 9 pounds could slash levels by up to 8 points in just a few weeks. In a 2013 University of Scranton study of 100 overweight people with high blood pressure, 39 percent of those who lost 10 to 15 percent of their body weight were able to work with their doctors to reduce their blood pressure medications.[13]

How weight loss helps: Getting rid of extra body fat promotes healthy BP in several important ways. Being overweight prompts your body to ramp up blood volume simply to ensure that oxygen and nutrients are supplied to your body fat stores. Trimming the fat reduces blood volume, automatically lowering blood pressure.[14] Extra fat stored in your midsection can also put extra pressure directly on your kidneys (even though they're located further up your torso), interfering with their ability to siphon off extra sodium.[15] Losing weight and blasting visceral fat—the deep belly fat that packs around your organs—also resets the delicate interplay of enzymes and hormones that regulate blood pressure. Being overweight boosts levels of pressure-raising compounds, including angiotensinogen, renin, aldosterone, and angiotensin converting enzyme. Losing weight lowers them, Columbia University heart experts report.[16] It also helps your kidneys send more sodium out of your body. And with less belly fat on board, your arteries get a break from inflammation-boosting compounds that make artery walls stiff.[17]

Increased waist circumference, due to belly fat, is associated with a multitude of complex hormonal mechanisms. The end result can be a decreased ability to metabolize sugars, leading to insulin resistance, high blood pressure, increased clotting, and inflammation. Having belly fat is an independent risk factor for the development of cardiovascular disease.

Strategy: Interval Walks

Exercise mows down rising BP levels even if you don't lose weight.[18] In fact, giving your walking shoes a workout could lower your blood pressure 8 to 10 points, notes the American Heart Association.[19] Boosting fitness, experts say, could wipe out 21 percent of hypertension![20]

The Lower Your Blood Pressure Naturally plan takes advantage of the latest research-proven ways to get more BP benefits from shorter, more convenient routines. Three days a week, you'll do a 20-minute interval walk that alternates bursts of moderate- and faster-paced movement.

Pushing the pace has the power to squash high BP as well as or better than sticking with longer, steady-paced strolls all the time, research shows.[21] When 88 Norwegians with high blood pressure did interval routines or steady-speed routines three times a week for a Norwegian University of Science and Technology study, researchers found that the interval group lowered systolic pressure an extra 7.5 points and diastolic pressure an extra 4.5 points.[22]

Interval walks work for almost everyone because you only have to speed up to a point that's challenging yet safe and comfortable for you. Adults in their forties, fifties, sixties,[23] and seventies; people recovering from heart surgery;[24] and those with heart failure[25] have all gotten benefits.

The effects go beyond BP, addressing other health and weight concerns faced by many people with elevated blood pressure. Intervals help you burn

---

No Time? Break It Up!

You'll take a steady-paced, 30-minute walk 3 days a week on this plan, but there's no need to set aside a full 30 minutes at once. Breaking these strolls up into two 15-minute chunks or even three 10-minute chunks throughout the day is even better for your blood pressure. New research shows that exercising for a few minutes throughout the day keeps pressure levels as low as one long exercise session and also provides more protection against brief BP spikes that damage arteries.[26]

---

more calories[27] and body fat,[28] become fitter faster, and keep your metabolism elevated (which also burns more calories) for up to 2½ hours[29] after a session. This type of exercise also enhances blood sugar processing, raises levels of heart-protecting HDL[30] cholesterol, and protects against heart disease.

How interval walks help: Increasing exercise intensity for 1 to 2 minutes at a time, then giving yourself a break by downshifting to a slower pace, boosts levels of artery-relaxing nitric oxide in blood vessels by 36 percent, something steady-state routines didn't do in one Brazilian study. Interval workouts also reduce levels of the heart-pounding stress hormone norepinephrine further, researchers report.[31]

Strategy: Strength Training

Pick up those dumbbells! Whether your chosen weights are ultralight or a bit heavier, hefting them twice a week—as you will on this plan—can make your muscles, arteries, and heart younger. Evidence that strength training promotes healthier blood pressure began emerging as early as the 1980s, when a big Massachusetts study of 1,600 women and men found that working out as little as twice a week could lower numbers up to 5 points.[32]

Newer research confirms the benefits. In a 2013 report that reviewed 25 muscle-building studies, the American Heart Association concluded that strength training can, indeed, lower systolic pressure by up to 4.6 points and

---

Is It Safe?

Interval workouts at a comfortable pace and strength training with weights that are right for you are safe exercise choices for most people. However, it's wise to check with your doctor before beginning to exercise if you haven't exercised lately, are overweight, have high blood pressure, or have a combination of heart disease risk factors (including high blood pressure, high cholesterol, diabetes, obesity, smoking, or a family history of heart disease). Check, too, if you have a strong family history of heart disease but don't know what your own risk is.

---

diastolic pressure by up to 4 points.[33] And in one 2012 Brazilian study of men with hypertension, strength training for 12 weeks reduced their numbers by 12 to 16 points and maintained their new, lower BP when researchers checked back a month later.[34]

Strength training can reverse the muscle loss that begins in our midthirties. We lose 2 percent or more every decade, enough to slow metabolism and pack on extra pounds because muscle burns more calories than fat around the clock.[35] Studies show that you can add 3 pounds of lean, calorie-torching muscle in 2½ months of strength training and lose 3.7 pounds of fat at the same time.[36] Muscle mass essentially allows the body to burn calories, even while you are sleeping.

How strength training helps: Revving up your body's natural ability to burn fat can help you lose weight and keep it off. Beyond that, experts aren't certain how strength training helps tame high blood pressure. Researchers suspect it may restore suppleness to arteries. If you have high blood pressure, choose lighter weights for the strength-training routine in this plan; working out with heavy weights could increase your blood pressure.

Strategy: Yoga

University of Pennsylvania researchers recently announced that a yoga practice reduced blood pressure readings by 3 points. In their study, 58 women and men performed a soothing routine two to three times a week or followed a special diet. The yogis got better BP results. A 2009 study by the same researchers found that long-held gentle poses and breathing exercises reduced systolic and diastolic pressure 5 points. For that study, yoga beginners did a simple 25-minute routine twice a week for 12 weeks.[37]

In the past, most evidence that yoga has a place in preventing or easing high BP has come from smaller studies that found big benefits but also contained big flaws that cast doubt on their findings. For example, in a 2005 study from Thailand, 27 people with hypertension who practiced yoga for 8 weeks reduced their BP levels by up to 24 points, but that report didn't say how blood pressure was monitored. But new, well-designed studies add new authority to yoga's role in lowering BP. "It looks very promising that yoga might be a useful therapy for patients with mild-to-moderate hypertension who want to avoid using medication. This could also be used as an adjunct to other lifestyle modifications," the lead researcher of the University of Pennsylvania study told the news media.[38]

How yoga helps: This movement-based mind-body therapy seems to work by reducing stress. That's crucial in our crazy-busy lives. Stopping tension with a period of deep calm turns off stress hormones, and the breathing techniques associated with yoga allow tight arteries to relax. Your cardiovascular system gets a break. And if you bust stress regularly, you're also teaching yourself how to get back to a state of relaxation easily and quickly. That's better for your blood pressure, your heart, and your whole being. Yoga as a stress management tool can decrease the release of stress hormones and inflammation.

Strategy: Meditation

Like yoga, meditation is attracting a growing number of fans among alternative medicine practitioners, conventional doctors, and those who use therapies from both worlds to help knock down high blood pressure. On this plan, you'll enjoy a "taste" of meditation: a 5-minute, do-anywhere breathing exercise designed to help you feel calm and centered.

Most evidence for meditation comes from studies of Transcendental Meditation (TM), which uses a repeated word or phrase—a mantra—to help meditators turn off ever-whirling thoughts and simply *be*. In two studies involving 143 people with high blood pressure, those who practiced TM daily for 3 months or more reduced their blood pressure numbers by 3 to 6 points. And when 298 college students tried TM, researchers found that those at high risk for developing high blood pressure (they were overweight, had prehypertension, or had family members with hypertension) saw their numbers improve. In a longer study, 201 people at risk for hypertension who practiced TM for 5 years were 48 percent less likely to have a heart attack or stroke than those who didn't meditate.[39]

These studies are important. But we think that any stress-reducing, meditative activity you enjoy—whether it's a few minutes of deep breathing, going out dancing, walking in your favorite park, or gardening—will have blood pressure benefits.

How meditation helps: This technique may soothe your sympathetic nervous system—which revs up blood pressure during stressful times—and trigger the pressure-lowering effects of your calm-and-serene parasympathetic nervous system. Again, slowing respiration leads to dilatation of the arteries. And when the parasympathetic nervous system is activated, heart rate decreases and blood pressure spikes that can occur with emotional upset or physical exertion are reduced.

Strategy: Blood Pressure Monitoring

The final member of the Lower Your Blood Pressure Naturally synergy team caught us by surprise. When we gave our test panelists home blood pressure monitors and asked them to track their numbers daily, we were just curious to see how the plan was working. But we quickly realized that home monitoring made the plan more effective.

Checking your own blood pressure can help you get better BP numbers for several reasons. You'll stay motivated when you see good results and get back on track quickly if you slip up and see your numbers rise. And simply checking every day and writing down your numbers will help you stay accountable. The American Heart Association recommends home monitoring for most people with hypertension or prehypertension and for those at high risk for high blood pressure.

And research confirms the benefits of self-checks. Doctors at Tufts Medical Center in Boston reviewed 52 blood pressure studies that included home monitoring. They found that keeping up with levels at home translated into a 3.9-point drop in systolic blood pressure and a 2.4-point drop in diastolic pressure. All that, just from switching on one of those nifty devices and putting it to use up to three or more times a day.[40]

How home monitoring helps: Accountability is one of the most powerful tools you can deploy for changing habits and making changes stick. Since you can't see or feel high blood pressure, home monitoring is the one way to know that your healthy lifestyle changes are working. In Chapter 17, you'll find advice on how often to check your blood pressure and how to take an accurate reading, along with a log to track your results.

Success Story: *Penny Boos*

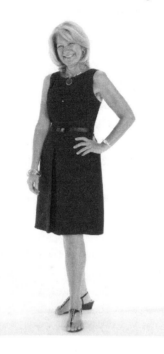

AGE: 55

HEIGHT: 5'6"

BLOOD PRESSURE IMPROVEMENT:
Penny's systolic pressure dropped
26 points and her diastolic pressure
dropped 13 points in 4 weeks.

POUNDS LOST: 2

Midlife women do have heart attacks,
and Penny Boos knows this firsthand.
"I had a heart attack last year," she says.
"I always had low blood pressure, but it
went up in my forties and just never
came down. I started with one blood
pressure pill, then my doctor added
another and another. If you need medication, that's fine. It can really help. But
it shouldn't be all you do. This plan has
shown me that by changing what I eat and being consistent with exercise, I
can keep my blood pressure down in a way that really helps my health."

In fact, Penny reduced her blood pressure from a high of 150/80 to a
healthy 124/67. She had already lost 15 pounds before she started the plan.
"I was hoping to lose just a little more weight," she says. "I did!" When she
weighed herself at home after completing the plan, she had lost 5 pounds
according to her scale.

"I've also lost 3 inches from my waist. I've gone from a size 12 to a size 10
and sometimes even wear a size 8. My boss and my husband both say they
can't believe the difference. I've had to go shopping for new clothes and
given away a lot of things that are now too big for me. I love it!"

She's experienced the dramatic, direct links between exercise, diet, and
heart health—in both directions. "I was feeling kind of depressed and
anxious and stopped exercising for about 6 to 9 months before my heart
attack," she notes. "Afterward, I told myself that I better start walking. But

I wasn't consistent until I started the plan. Now I meet my boss at 6:30 in the morning to take a power walk, shower at the company gym, and go to work."

Penny noticed a change in her blood pressure on the second day of the plan. "I think it was because I had reduced my sodium intake and increased the minerals," she says. "When I saw the drop in my blood pressure, I thought my monitor was broken. I used Bryon's monitor and confirmed that the change was real."

Recently, she and her husband, Bryon (who also followed the plan and lowered his blood pressure and weight), had a revelation while food shopping. "I turned to Bryon and said, 'You notice how our shopping habits have changed? We stay in one section of the store now—where the produce and the dairy products are!' And we'll continue to shop and eat this way."

The couple discovered that prepping ingredients ahead of time made putting together plan meals quick and easy. "We decided to eat spinach instead of kale. We just liked the flavor more," she says. "At one point, I bought nine containers of spinach on sale, blanched it in 2-cup servings, drained it on paper towels, and froze it. I also freeze leftover fruit and even mashed avocado to use later on. It's really easy to just toss all of the frozen ingredients into the blender and make a smoothie."

Penny thought the meals tasted great. "I would get so excited about the food," she says. "With Bryon working so much and doing shift work at times, I would do a lot of the cooking. I was always taking pictures with my phone and sending them to him: 'Here's the dinner waiting for you,' 'Here's the breakfast waiting for you.' When I made the Corn Tortilla Pizzas (page 120), I put little smiley faces on them with cherry tomatoes. That's exactly how I felt about the plan."

CHAPTER 6

Prep for Success

Ready to jump in and lower your blood pressure naturally? High blood pressure is a serious condition that deserves serious attention—at home and from your health care practitioner. Follow these steps to get the most from the plan.

Know your blood pressure. If you haven't had a blood pressure check in the past 2 years, schedule one with your doctor. It's important to know where you stand and to get immediate help from pressure-lowering medications if your readings are high. Remember that medication can't take the place of the healthy changes you'll make on this plan; together, though, they can help keep your BP lower and healthier than drugs alone can. (Sometimes medications can be a bridge of safety while you are getting your blood pressure under control.

Talk with your doctor about your medications. Some people may be able to reduce their doses or even take fewer drugs once their BP comes down and stays down. However, never change the dose or stop taking your medications without the advice or prior approval of your doctor. If you take blood pressure drugs now, keep it up. Tell your doctor you are starting a healthy lifestyle program that will make it easier for you to control your blood pressure, and ask what you should do if you notice your blood pressure numbers are coming down. The daily monitoring we recommend doing on this plan will give you invaluable information that you and your doctor can use to make decisions about your care.

Get your doctor's okay for exercise. If you have high blood pressure, are over age 50, haven't exercised much in the past few months, are overweight, or have a strong family history of heart disease but don't know your own risk, get your doctor's approval before doing the workout in this plan. If you have any symptoms of chest pain or pressure, shortness of breath, jaw pain, back pain, or flulike symptoms with fatigue (especially with exertion), discuss them with your doctor. These subtle signs might indicate that something is wrong with your heart, and you might need a more thorough investigation before starting an exercise program. While every element of this plan is proven to help with blood pressure, some may not be right for you. Talk with your doctor about the best pace for interval walks, about strength training (how light or heavy your weights should be, if there are any moves you should skip), and about the yoga routines (certain moves could raise blood pressure for some people). Bring this book along so your doctor can see all of the details.

Know what to do if your blood pressure drops too far. Call your doctor if your systolic blood pressure—the top or first number in your reading—falls below 100. If you start feeling light-headed, dizzy, or very fatigued, you should also call your doctor. These symptoms can be a sign of low blood pressure as well.

Invest in a home blood pressure monitor and become a monitoring "pro." Checking your blood pressure once or twice a day—more if your doctor recommends it—can help you stay on track and get better results. You can find inexpensive home blood pressure monitors at drugstores and discount retailers. Buy one in advance and learn how to use it. To get the most accurate reading, follow the expert advice about blood pressure logging in Chapter 17.

Stock your kitchen. Read about Phase 1 of the eating plan in Chapter 8. Then, create a shopping list a few days before you begin the plan. Having all the ingredients that you'll need on hand will make meal prep a breeze. And consider precooking some ingredients, like quinoa and sweet potatoes, for fast meals.

Get your gear. Are your walking shoes, socks, and sweatpants ready? Do you have the right weights and a yoga mat? Turn to Chapters 11, 12, and 13 to find out what you'll need for workouts. If you don't own sneakers, go buy them. It is well worth the investment.

Part II

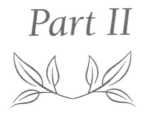

The
Power Mineral Diet

At a Glance:
The Eating Plan

Phase 1

Week 1: Meet the Power Foods!

For the first week of the Lower Your Blood Pressure Naturally plan, you'll enjoy delicious meals built with just 13 Power Foods, which are naturally low in sodium and calories, yet rich in the blood pressure–friendly Power Minerals calcium, magnesium, and potassium. You'll use these 13 foods—pork tenderloin, white beans, fat-free yogurt, tilapia, kiwifruit, peaches (or nectarines), bananas, kale, red bell peppers, broccoli, quinoa, sweet potato, and avocado—along with basic kitchen staples, such as olive oil and garlic, to turn out tasty breakfasts, lunches, and dinners. You'll also start using our five customized seasoning blends to flavor your meals without an overload of pressure-boosting salt.

Sample meals: Sweet Potato Hash (page 90), Red Bell Pepper Stuffed with Pork and Quinoa (page 100), Creamy Banana Smoothie (page 89), Peaches and Cream Hot Quinoa Cereal (page 87)

What to do: Eat four satisfying meals a day! Always choose one meal from our Phase 1 breakfast options to ensure optimal levels of pressure-lowering minerals. Your other three daily meal choices can come from Phase 1 lunch and dinner options or from Phase 1 breakfast options.

Nutrition facts: A day of Phase 1 meals provides 1,300 to 1,350 calories, 2,300 milligrams of sodium or less, 1,200 milligrams of calcium, 420 milligrams of magnesium, and 4,700 milligrams of potassium. And these meals deliver plenty of heart-healthy and satisfying fiber, the recommended levels of lean protein and good fats, and a full range of important vitamins, minerals, and micronutrients.

Benefits: With a lower calorie count, Phase 1 jump-starts weight loss (including shedding belly fat). And the infusion of Power Minerals means you may begin seeing positive changes in your blood pressure before the week is over. Many of our test panelists did!

Phase 2

Weeks 2 to 6: Enjoy Four Daily Meals plus a Smoothie or Dessert!

In Phase 2, Weeks 2 through 6 of the plan, you'll branch out by enjoying a wider variety of mineral-rich foods and a delicious daily addition: a dessert or smoothie. You'll choose from a broader selection of proteins, fruits, vegetables, whole grains, good fats, and dairy foods. Ingredients you'll savor include cheese, shrimp, spinach, chicken, mushrooms, whole grain bread, white potatoes, bulgur, black beans, and more. Many meals as well as smoothies and sweet treats still feature our 13 original Power Foods.

Sample meals, desserts, and smoothies: Tex-Mex Black Bean and Bulgur Burger (page 122), Corn Tortilla Pizzas (page 120), Garlic-Ginger Tofu Stir-Fry (page 116), Veggie and Cheddar Frittata (page 113), Peach-Almond Ice Cream Cup (page 127), Peanut Butter–Banana Frozen Yogurt (page 129), Orange-Carrot Creamsicle Smoothie (page 125), Berries and Cream Smoothie (page 126)

What to do: Choose four meals plus a smoothie or dessert every day. For optimal mineral intake, each day choose one Phase 1 meal (a breakfast, lunch, or dinner) and three Phase 2 meals (from the breakfast, lunch, or dinner options). To get the most minerals, have a smoothie four times a week and a dessert three times a week.

Nutrition facts: A day of Phase 2 eating provides 1,500 to 1,550 calories, 2,300 milligrams of sodium or less, 1,200 milligrams of calcium, 420 milligrams of magnesium, and 4,700 milligrams of potassium. You also get all of the fiber, lean protein, good fats, and other nutrients—vitamins, minerals, micronutrients—essential for great health.

Benefits: Calorie-controlled portions make it easy to keep on losing pounds without counting calories. And you'll continue to take in all of the calcium, magnesium, and potassium your body needs for better blood pressure regulation.

Success Story: Kristi Oblas

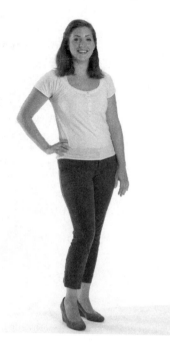

AGE: 26

HEIGHT: 5'4½"

BLOOD PRESSURE IMPROVEMENT:
Kristi's systolic pressure fell 13 points,
and her diastolic pressure fell 7 points.

INCHES LOST: 2 from her waist,
1½ from her hips

Already a slim 144 pounds, Kristi lost body fat as she lowered her blood pressure on this plan. "My pants fit better. I like seeing this change," she says. Even better: Her blood pressure fell from a high of 143/93 to a healthier 130/86. "My blood pressure went down to a more acceptable level, which was my main goal," she notes.

Kristi tested out the plan along with her husband, David Oblas. "I think the foods in the plan helped the most to make our blood pressure levels decline," she says. "The Phase 1 recipes were full of foods packed with those essential minerals that aid in the lowering of blood pressure. I enjoyed eating the peaches, kiwis, pork, sweet potatoes, quinoa, bell peppers, Greek yogurt (in Phase 2), bananas, and tilapia. We are still pretty consistent with incorporating these foods into our daily meals. When I plan meals, I always try to make sure to include them."

The couple says their blood pressure levels responded quickly to their new way of eating. "We saw results the next day," she notes. "I was quite surprised with how quickly our blood pressures went down to normal levels. I shared my results with friends and family. They were surprised that just eating the right kinds of food could help. I actually suggested my mom talk to her doctor and try out the plan to lower her blood pressure."

In addition to the eating plan, Kristi made time for the 5-minute meditation every day. "I found it helped me relax," she says. "I felt the stress released from my body."

CHAPTER 7

Eating Plan FAQs

Wondering what you can drink, whether the plan will work if you have a food intolerance, or how to make meal prep easier? Before you start the plan, read this chapter to find the answers to these and many more questions.

Q: What can I drink on the plan?

A: We recommend water or unsweetened herbal tea (hot or iced) with a spritz of lemon or lime. A cup of coffee or caffeinated tea at breakfast is fine. Skip alcohol during the plan—it just adds extra calories and can make sticking with healthy eating choices more challenging.

Q: Why is there salt in some of the recipes?

A: The plan keeps your daily sodium intake below 2,300 milligrams a day, the level recommended for most Americans by the Centers for Disease Control and Prevention. More than 75 percent of the sodium in the American diet comes from restaurant meals, processed foods, and fast food. By removing these, this eating plan gives you some leeway to use very small amounts of added sodium in the best way possible: as a flavor enhancer that won't raise your blood pressure.

Q: I'm not "salt sensitive," so can I have more salt?

A: No. The level of sodium in this plan is carefully balanced with the levels of calcium, potassium, and magnesium, and all are balanced with calorie counts that will help you lose weight. Adding extra sodium may render the three Power Minerals less effective, making it more difficult for your body to maintain healthy blood pressure. Your body can store sodium, for example, but it cannot store potassium. We've kept sodium at an enjoyable yet moderately low level so that you get enough for healthy functioning and tasty food and so that the Power Minerals work optimally. Although people who are salt sensitive have an increase in blood pressure when they eat salt, this diet is meant to recalibrate the body for efficient metabolism of the minerals and nutrients found in the chosen foods.

Q: How can I further reduce the sodium in this plan?

A: Eliminate the small amounts of salt used in some recipes. Be sure to use no-salt-added canned beans and to choose breads with the lowest sodium content. Use low-sodium cheeses (Swiss, for example) or choose recipes that do not call for cheese.

Q: I'm cooking for two or more people. How can I adjust the recipes?

A: Almost every recipe in Phase 1 and Phase 2 makes one serving; a few make two servings. Check the recipe you'd like to make and just multiply the ingredient quantities by the number of servings you need. A calculator may come in handy.

Q: Can I cook ahead for easier meal preparation?

A: Yes. Several recipes call for cooked quinoa or bulgur, two grains you can cook ahead of time and refrigerate for about 4 days or freeze (in single-portion servings) for even longer. Several recipes call for pork tenderloin, cooked and cut into bite-size chunks, such as Pork Stir-Fry with Quinoa (page 92) and Red Bell Pepper Stuffed with Pork and Quinoa (page 100). You'll save time by roasting a larger tenderloin in advance and using it for these recipes.

Q: Several recipes call for no-salt-added canned white beans. What if I can't find them or I want to use dried beans?

A: You can substitute either. If you cannot find no-salt-added canned beans, look for reduced-sodium beans or just use regular canned beans and rinse well. Dump the beans into a strainer and rinse under cool water until the water running out of the beans is clear. You can remove about 50 percent of the added sodium this way. If you'd like to use dried beans, follow the directions on the bag and make them in advance. Cook them without added salt and store in the refrigerator for up to 5 days.

Q: Several recipes call for part of a banana, avocado, tomato, or peach. What can I do with the rest so that it doesn't go to waste?

A: Drop unused pieces of cut fruit into a resealable plastic freezer bag and freeze to use later in a smoothie. Cover unused cut tomato with plastic wrap and refrigerate. Or, instead of slicing a regular tomato, use a few cherry tomatoes, halved. When a recipe calls for part of an avocado, keep the rest from turning brown by leaving the pit in place and rubbing the exposed flesh with lemon or lime juice. Put the avocado in a plastic bag; it will keep in the refrigerator for up to 2 days. You could also try the thrifty shortcut one test panelist developed: She mashed together extra banana and avocado and froze single-serving portions to use later in Phase 1 breakfasts.

Q: I'm lactose intolerant. Can I adjust the plan to avoid using regular milk?

A: Absolutely. Stay comfortable by using lactose-free milk. You can also take tablets or use drops containing the enzyme that breaks down lactose so that your body can digest milk more easily. You will probably have no trouble digesting the yogurt in this plan. The lactose (milk sugar) in this fermented food has already been broken down by friendly bacteria. If you prefer, choose an alternative milk—like those made from soy, almonds, or rice—that's calcium fortified and close to 90 calories per cup.

Q: I avoid wheat products because I'm gluten intolerant. Is there much wheat in this plan?

A: There's no wheat in Phase 1. For the first week of the plan, the only grain you'll eat is gluten-free quinoa. In Phase 2, some gluten-containing grain products, such as bulgur, are introduced. But with so many recipes to choose from, you can easily avoid gluten. Or substitute gluten-free grains. For example, use quinoa or brown rice in place of bulgur. Instead of whole grain wheat bread, choose a gluten-free bread that you enjoy. If you are extremely sensitive to gluten, you may be concerned about oats as well. While oats do not contain gluten, this grain may come in contact with gluten during processing. Use quinoa instead or oats that have not been contaminated with gluten. Companies such as Bob's Red Mill, Cream Hill Estates, GF Harvest, Avena Foods (Only Oats), Legacy Valley, and Gifts of Nature offer these oat products.

Q: I'm a vegetarian. Can I follow this plan?

A: Absolutely. Many of the Lower Your Blood Pressure Naturally meals are meatless. Meals that feature produce, fat-free dairy products, nuts, and beans deliver significant amounts of calcium, magnesium, and potassium. If you'd like, you can use tofu in many Phase 1 recipes that call for pork tenderloin or tilapia.

Q: What about vegans? How can someone who doesn't eat any animal products follow this diet?

A: Easily! Start with meals that don't include fish or meat. Swap out milk and yogurt made with cow's milk for calcium-fortified versions made with a dairy alternative, like soy milk. In Phase 2, replace mozzarella or Cheddar cheese with low-sodium soy cheese.

Q: Can I eat out?

A: Eat at home (if possible) during Phase 1 so that you get the full combination of Power Minerals. Starting in Week 2, it's fine to eat an occasional meal away from home, following the guidelines and suggestions in Chapter 10. You'll find tips and selected items from the menus of dozens of fast-food and casual dining chains. We've identified low-sodium, reduced-calorie options that deliver at least some of the Power Minerals you need at each meal.

Q: I don't always have time to cook. Are there no-cook ways to follow the plan?

A: Yes! Even though most processed and packaged foods are too high in sodium, we've found a few that are low enough to work on this plan. We've combined them with easy-to-toss-together sides that bump up the mineral content of these fast meals. In Chapter 10, you'll find these options along with a shopping list of side-dish foods to keep on hand.

Q: Is it okay to use salt substitutes?

A: The American Heart Association suggests talking with your doctor before using a salt substitute. "Lite" salt is about a 50-50 blend with potassium chloride, and salt-free substitutes can be 100 percent potassium chloride. Salt substitutes can be harmful for people with diabetes or kidney disease; those who have had a blocked urinary flow; or those taking a potassium-sparing diuretic, an ACE inhibitor, or an angiotensin II receptor blocker. The safest way to substitute for salt is by using spices instead. Try the spice blends in Chapter 8.

Q: Should I take vitamin or mineral supplements on the plan?

A: This is not a simple answer, as many recent studies have shown no benefit to many of the common vitamin supplements. This plan provides 100 percent of the calcium, magnesium, and potassium you need every day. It also provides a full range of vitamins and other minerals you need to stay healthy. That said, if you feel you want to take a multivitamin, talk with your doctor about the pros and cons.

Q: I have diabetes. Is this eating plan right for me?

A: Review the plan with your doctor, a registered dietitian, or a certified diabetes educator to be sure the carbohydrate levels are right for you. Fiber and whole grains are an important part of a diabetic diet, and minimizing saturated fats is important as well. The good fats, lean protein, and fiber in this plan help keep your blood sugar lower and steadier. And over time, weight loss on the plan can help your body become more sensitive to signals from insulin, the hormone that tells cells to absorb blood sugar.

Q: Will this plan help my high cholesterol?

A: Many elements of this heart-healthy eating plan can also rebalance your blood fats. The good fats in the plan can help support healthy levels of helpful HDL cholesterol, while the soluble fiber can help whisk heart-threatening LDLs out of your body. Weight loss will also help lower your LDL cholesterol. A diet high in whole grains, low in saturated fats, and high in omega-3s has been shown to reduce LDLs, increase HDLs, and stabilize triglycerides.

Q: How do I figure out how much food to buy?

A: We have included worksheets and shopping lists in Chapters 8 and 9 to help you with meal planning and shopping. A few days in advance, sit down and choose your meals for the coming week and input them into the appropriate menu planning worksheet. Then, tally up the amounts of each food you'll need on the shopping lists provided (there is one for Phase 1 and another for Phase 2). Take them with you to the store to make shopping a snap. Don't forget to check your supply of pantry staples as well.

Q: What if I'm hungry on the plan?

A: If you're a large man or an extremely active man or woman, you may need extra calories. If you feel hungry after a few days on the plan, add more calories by having a cup of fat-free plain yogurt with fruit or by increasing the size of one of your meals by an extra 50 percent.

CHAPTER 8

Phase 1: The Power Mineral Jump-Start

For the next 7 days, your food life will be very simple—and very powerful. Phase 1 of the Lower Your Blood Pressure Naturally plan introduces you to 13 amazing Power Foods rich in blood pressure-regulating Power Minerals: calcium, magnesium, and potassium. With the addition of just a few everyday kitchen staples, your meals will be made entirely from these versatile and delicious foods.

Without counting calories or fat grams, you'll start losing weight. Without tracking milligrams of sodium, your consumption of salt will fall to a healthy and sustainable level. Without tallying quantities, you'll bump up your mineral intake to reach recommended daily levels that few Americans ever reach. The result: You'll reset your body chemistry for optimal blood pressure control while your tastebuds are having a wonderful adventure. Our test panelists loved the foods they discovered in Phase 1 and continued to make them an important part of their meals long after the program ended.

And that's exactly the purpose of Phase 1: To give you plenty of new ways to use BP Power Foods every day so that eating them regularly—and flooding your body with the right nutrients for heart health—becomes your new normal. At the same time, you'll notice your tastebuds waking up as they anticipate and savor all of the flavors in food that get hidden by the high levels of salt most of us scarf down every day.

Stocking Your Kitchen for Phase 1

All meals in Phase 1 are made with our 13 mineral-rich Power Foods plus some basic kitchen staples (listed on the next page). The quantity of each food that you'll need will vary depending on which meals you choose. Quantities will also vary depending on whether you're cooking for one, two, or more people.

To figure out how much food to buy for Phase 1, choose your meals in advance. Check the ingredients list at the top of each recipe and add up how much of each Power Food you'll need for the week. Write the number beside each food below to make shopping a breeze.

POWER FOOD SHOPPING LIST

FOOD	QUANTITY YOU'LL NEED
Avocados	
Bananas	
Broccoli	
Kale	
Kiwifruit	
Peaches/nectarines (you can also choose frozen peach slices or canned peach slices in juice or light syrup)	
Pork tenderloin	
Quinoa (sold in the grains aisle or with "natural" foods)	
Red bell peppers	
Sweet potatoes	
Tilapia fillets	
White beans (no-salt-added canned, or dry)	
Fat-free plain yogurt	

KITCHEN STAPLES

Phase 1 recipes also call for some basic staples that you probably have on hand. These are:

- Olive oil
- Canola oil
- Vinegar
- Flour
- Onion
- Garlic
- Reduced-sodium chicken broth
- Kosher salt or coarse sea salt (you'll get the same salty flavor with a little less sodium)
- Dried herbs and spices (see list below)
- Lemons and limes
- Fat-free milk or soy milk

Note: To make the signature spice blends (the recipes start on page 84) used throughout the 6 weeks of the plan, you will need a variety of dried herbs and spices as well as a few other ingredients. However, we recommend reading the recipes first to choose which you would like to make. You can also use other no-salt seasoning blends in the recipes.

To make all five spice blends, you will need:

dried basil	cumin seeds	onion powder
ground black pepper	curry powder	dried oregano
black peppercorns	fennel seeds	paprika
brown sugar	garlic powder	ground red pepper
chili powder	ground ginger	red-pepper flakes
ground cinnamon	hazelnuts	dried rosemary
ground coriander	kosher salt	sesame seeds
coriander seeds	dried marjoram	dried thyme
ground cumin	dried mint	ground turmeric

Phase 1 Eating

Choose four meals every day and make sure at least one is a Phase 1 break-fast. A day of Phase 1 meals provides 1,300 to 1,350 calories; 2,300 milli-grams or less sodium; 1,200 milligrams calcium; 420 milligrams magnesium; and 4,700 milligrams potassium. All recipes in this book are designed to yield one serving unless otherwise noted.

Spice Blend Recipes

You will use these low-salt and no-salt blends throughout Phases 1 and 2. They're a delicious way to bring out natural flavors without an overload of sodium.

Dukkah

This Middle Eastern nut and spice mix is gaining a following in the United States. It's delicious!

Makes ½ cup / Serving size = 1 tablespoon

¼	cup hazelnuts	½	tablespoon black peppercorns
2	tablespoons coriander seeds	½	teaspoon fennel seeds
1½	tablespoons sesame seeds	½	teaspoon dried mint
1	tablespoon cumin seeds	¼	teaspoon kosher salt

1. In a heavy skillet over high heat, toast the hazelnuts for 3 minutes, or until the nuts become fragrant, being careful not to burn them. Transfer the hazelnuts to a small bowl, then repeat this process with the coriander seeds, sesame seeds, cumin seeds, peppercorns, and fennel seeds.

2. When the nuts and seeds are cooled, add the mint and salt. Using a mortar and pestle or the back of a spoon, crush the mixture until you have a coarse blend. Or place in a food processor and pulse a few times until you reach the desired coarse consistency.

3. Transfer the mixture to an airtight container and store in a cool place. This spice blend is great sprinkled on meats, cooked vegetables, and veg-etarian main dishes.

PER SERVING: 41 calories, 75 mg sodium

Tex-Mex Spice Blend

Makes approximately ¼ cup / Serving size = 1 teaspoon

6   teaspoons chili powder

5   teaspoons ground cumin

½   teaspoon kosher salt

½   teaspoon garlic powder

½   teaspoon onion powder

⅛   teaspoon ground black pepper

⅛   teaspoon ground red pepper (optional)

In a small bowl, mix all of the ingredients together. Store in an airtight container in a cool place. Use as a spice rub on chicken, pork, fish, or beef; sprinkle over veggies; or add to sauces and dips for additional flavor.

PER SERVING: 72 mg sodium

Indian Spice Blend

Makes approximately 6 tablespoons / Serving size = 1 teaspoon

3   tablespoons curry powder

1   teaspoon kosher salt

2   teaspoons red-pepper flakes

1½ teaspoons ground cumin

1½ teaspoons ground coriander

1½ teaspoons dried mint

1   teaspoon ground turmeric

1   teaspoon ground ginger

In a small bowl, mix all of the ingredients together. Store in an airtight container in a cool place. Use as a spice rub on chicken, pork, fish, or beef; sprinkle over veggies; or add to sauces and dips for additional flavor.

PER SERVING: 127 mg sodium

Italian Spice Blend

Makes approximately ¾ cup / Serving size = 1 teaspoon

3 tablespoons dried basil

3 tablespoons dried oregano

2½ tablespoons dried parsley

2 tablespoons dried marjoram

1 teaspoon garlic powder

1 teaspoon dried thyme

1 teaspoon dried rosemary

¼ teaspoon ground black pepper

¼ teaspoon red-pepper flakes (optional)

In a small bowl, mix all of the ingredients together. Store in an airtight container in a cool place. Use as a seasoning on chicken, pork, fish, or beef or to add flavor to sauces or dips.

PER SERVING: <1 mg sodium

BBQ Rub

Makes 10 tablespoons / Serving size = 1 teaspoon

2 tablespoons brown sugar

2 tablespoons paprika

2 tablespoons chili powder

1 tablespoon ground black pepper

1 tablespoon garlic powder

1 tablespoon onion powder

2 teaspoons ground cinnamon

1 teaspoon ground red pepper (use more or less to adjust heat)

In a small bowl, mix all of the ingredients together. Store in an airtight container in a cool place.

PER SERVING: 10 mg sodium

Phase 1 Breakfasts

A hearty hot cereal. A fruity yogurt parfait. A creamy, sweet banana smoothie. And a trendy "green drink" brimming with nutrients that favor healthy blood pressure. In Phase 1, you'll wake up to these options for your morning meal. Every day this week, choose at least one Phase 1 breakfast as one of your four daily meals.

Peaches and Cream Hot Quinoa Cereal

3	tablespoons quinoa	½	cup sliced peaches
1	cup fat-free milk	¼	cup sliced banana
	Dash of vanilla extract	⅓	cup fat-free plain yogurt
	Sprinkle of ground cinnamon		

1. In a small pot, bring the quinoa, milk, vanilla, and cinnamon to a boil. Cover, reduce the heat to medium, and let simmer for 12 to 15 minutes, or until the quinoa is soft. (There may be a small amount of milk that hasn't been absorbed by the quinoa, but do not drain.)

2. Reduce the heat to low and add the peaches and banana and warm for 30 seconds.

3. Remove from the heat and stir in the yogurt.

TIME-SAVING HINT: *Cook extra quinoa in advance. In the morning, heat ¾ cup cooked quinoa with the milk and vanilla. Add the fruit, heat, and stir in the yogurt.*

PER SERVING: 310 calories, 19 g protein, 55 g carbohydrates, 3 g total fat, 0.5 g saturated fat, 4 g fiber, 168 mg sodium, 490 mg calcium, 1,050 mg potassium, 122 mg magnesium

Kiwi-Peach Yogurt Parfait

⅛ avocado

½ banana

1 cup fat-free plain yogurt

Ground cinnamon

1 kiwifruit, finely chopped

½ cup finely chopped peaches

In a small bowl, mash the avocado and banana into the yogurt. Stir in the cinnamon to taste. Layer with the kiwi and peaches.

FOOD STORAGE TIP: *Mash and freeze extra avocado and banana to use in future parfaits or in smoothies.*

PER SERVING: 306 calories, 17 g protein, 53 g carbohydrates, 5 g total fat, 1 g saturated fat, 7 g fiber, 193 mg sodium, 193 mg calcium, 1,341 mg potassium, 90 mg magnesium

Green Machine Smoothie

1 cup fat-free plain yogurt

½ cup kale (washed, coarsely chopped, and larger sections of stems removed)

½ banana

1 kiwifruit

⅛ avocado

Ice (optional)

In a blender, combine the yogurt, kale, banana, kiwi, and avocado. Blend until smooth. Add ice as needed for a frothier smoothie.

PER SERVING: 293 calories, 18 g protein, 49 g carbohydrates, 5 g total fat, 1 g saturated fat, 6 g fiber, 206 mg sodium, 570 mg calcium, 1,359 mg potassium, 99 mg magnesium

Creamy Banana Smoothie

1 frozen banana	Ground cinnamon (optional)
¾ cup fat-free plain yogurt	Ground nutmeg (optional)
½ cup fat-free milk	Ice (optional)
½ cooked sweet potato (with or without skin)	

In a blender, combine the banana, yogurt, milk, potato, cinnamon to taste (if using), and nutmeg to taste (if using). (Cinnamon and nutmeg add a sweet potato pie flavor.) Blend until smooth. Add ice as needed for a frothier smoothie.

TIME-SAVING HINT: *Bake or microwave the sweet potato in advance. Store in the refrigerator in a plastic bag or food container.*

PER SERVING: 307 calories, 17 g protein, 61 g carbohydrates, 1 g total fat, 0.5 g saturated fat, 5 g fiber, 215 mg sodium, 545 mg calcium, 1,256 mg potassium, 94 mg magnesium

Phase 1 Lunches and Dinners

In addition to breakfast, you get three lunch/dinner selections daily during Phase 1! Use your fourth meal as a hearty snack, or combine two meals for a double-size lunch or dinner if you're hungry. These meals incorporate our four Phase 1 proteins—yogurt, white beans, pork tenderloin, and tilapia—with the featured vegetables, fruits, starches, and good fat. You'll be surprised by the wide range of meals you can make with just a few simple, blood pressure–friendly ingredients. And that's part of the plan. We want you to discover lots of ways to use these important ingredients so that they'll always have a place in your repertoire as versatile, go-to foods.

All of these meals work as lunches or dinners. You'll probably discover, as many test panelists did, that cooking extra for dinner gives you leftovers to pack for an easy lunch the next day. Reminder: Every day this week, have four Phase 1 meals. One should be a breakfast. The other three can be lunches, dinners, or an additional breakfast choice.

Sweet Potato Hash

1   teaspoon olive oil

1   sweet potato with skin, finely chopped

¼   cup chopped onion

½   cup finely chopped red bell pepper

⅔   cup canned no-salt-added white beans, rinsed and drained

½   teaspoon BBQ Rub (page 86)

⅛   teaspoon salt

1. In a large skillet over medium-high heat, warm the oil. Cook the potato, stirring frequently, for 5 minutes, or until the flesh begins to soften and the sides are lightly browned.

2. Add the onion and pepper and cook for 3 minutes, or until the onion is golden and the pepper is soft.

3. Add the beans and BBQ Rub and cook for an additional 2 minutes, until heated through. Sprinkle with the salt before serving.

PER SERVING: 347 calories, 15 g protein, 62 g carbohydrates, 5 g total fat, 1 g saturated fat, 14 g fiber, 344 mg sodium, 165 mg calcium, 1,426 mg potassium, 119 mg magnesium

Twice-Baked Spiced Sweet Potato with Roasted Broccoli and Tilapia

1 sweet potato with skin

2 tablespoons fat-free plain yogurt

¾ teaspoon Indian Spice Blend, divided (page 85)

2 cups broccoli florets

1½ teaspoons olive oil

1 tilapia fillet (4 ounces)

Pinch of ground black pepper

¼ teaspoon garlic powder

1. Preheat the oven to 350°F. Line a baking sheet with foil.

2. Poke several holes in the potato and microwave on high power for 4 to 5 minutes, or until soft. Allow to cool slightly.

3. Halve the potato lengthwise and scrape out the flesh, leaving ¼" attached to the skin. In a small bowl, mash the removed flesh with the yogurt and ¼ teaspoon of the spice blend. Place the mixture back into each potato half.

4. In a medium bowl, toss the broccoli with the oil and lay it out on the baking sheet. Place the tilapia and the stuffed potato halves next to the broccoli.

5. Rub the remaining ½ teaspoon spice blend over the top of the tilapia. Sprinkle the pepper and garlic powder over the broccoli, tilapia, and potato halves.

6. Bake for 25 minutes, or until the broccoli is tender and the tilapia flakes easily.

PER SERVING: 357 calories, 32 g protein, 40 g carbohydrates, 10 g total fat, 2 g saturated fat, 9 g fiber, 279 mg sodium, 208 mg calcium, 1,566 mg potassium, 109 mg magnesium

Pork Stir-Fry with Quinoa

1 tablespoon lime juice

¼ teaspoon minced garlic

Pinch of ground black pepper

3 ounces pork tenderloin, cut into 1" cubes

1 teaspoon olive oil

⅓ cup sliced onion

⅓ cup sliced red bell pepper

½ cup chopped broccoli

1 cup chopped kale

⅛ teaspoon salt

2 teaspoons Dukkah spice mix (page 84)

½ cup cooked quinoa (prepared according to package directions)

1. In a medium bowl, whisk together the lime juice, garlic, and black pepper.

2. Place the pork in the lime juice mixture. Cover with plastic wrap and refrigerate for 5 to 10 minutes.

3. Remove the pork from the fridge and drain off the excess marinade. In a large skillet over medium-high heat, warm the oil. Cook the pork, stirring frequently, for 4 minutes, or until it turns white.

4. Add the onion, bell pepper, broccoli, and kale. Season with the salt and cook for 4 minutes, or until the pork is browned and the veggies are tender.

5. In a small bowl, stir the spice mix into the quinoa. Top with the pork stir-fry.

PER SERVING: 360 calories, 28 g protein, 40 g carbohydrates, 11 g total fat, 2 g saturated fat, 7 g fiber, 437 mg sodium, 178 mg calcium, 1,217 mg potassium, 149 mg magnesium

Kale Salad with Roasted Peaches, Spiced Yogurt-Avocado Dressing, and Tilapia

¼ cup fat-free plain yogurt

1 teaspoon Dukkah spice mix (page 84)

1 teaspoon lemon juice

¼ teaspoon minced garlic

¼ avocado, mashed

½ peach, sliced, or ½ cup canned (in juice) and drained, or frozen and thawed sliced peaches

½ teaspoon olive oil, divided

1 tilapia fillet (4 ounces)

⅛ teaspoon salt

Pinch of ground black pepper

2 cups chopped kale

⅓ cup finely chopped red bell pepper

1. Preheat the oven to 350°F.

2. In a medium bowl, whisk together the yogurt, spice mix, lemon juice, garlic, and avocado. Set aside.

3. In a small bowl, combine the peaches with ¼ teaspoon of the oil and set aside.

4. Place the tilapia in a baking pan and drizzle with the remaining ¼ teaspoon oil. Season with the salt and black pepper and bake for 15 minutes. Add the reserved peach mixture and bake for 10 minutes, or until the fish flakes easily.

5. Meanwhile, add the kale and bell pepper to the reserved dressing and toss.

6. To serve, top the kale with the roasted peaches and tilapia.

PER SERVING: 355 calories, 34 g protein, 30 g carbohydrates, 14 g total fat, 2 g saturated fat, 8 g fiber, 477 mg sodium, 357 mg calcium, 1,580 mg potassium, 134 mg magnesium

White Bean–Sweet Potato Patties over Kale Topped with Yogurt Sauce

3 tablespoons fat-free plain yogurt

1 teaspoon lemon juice

¼ teaspoon minced garlic

⅛ teaspoon salt

¾ teaspoon Indian Spice Blend, divided (page 85)

1 sweet potato

¼ cup canned no-salt-added white beans, rinsed and drained

¼ cup cooked quinoa (prepared according to package directions)

1 teaspoon olive oil

1½ cups chopped kale

¼ cup sliced onion

1. In a small bowl, whisk together the yogurt, lemon juice, garlic, salt, and ¼ teaspoon of the spice blend. Set aside.

2. Poke several holes in the potato and microwave on high power for 4 to 5 minutes, or until soft. Let cool slightly, halve lengthwise, and remove the flesh. Discard the skin.

3. In a medium bowl, mash the potato flesh with the beans until smooth. Stir in the quinoa and the remaining ½ teaspoon spice blend. Form into 2 patties, each ½" thick.

4. In a large skillet over medium-high heat, warm the oil. Cook the patties, kale, and onion for 4 minutes, or until the patties are browned on one side and the veggies are soft.

5. Flip the patties, stir the veggies, and cook for 3 minutes.

6. Serve the patties over the kale mixture, drizzled with the reserved yogurt sauce.

PER SERVING: 365 calories, 17 g protein, 64 g carbohydrates, 7 g total fat, 1 g saturated fat, 11 g fiber, 218 mg sodium, 356 mg calcium, 1,599 mg potassium, 157 mg magnesium

Garlicky Kale and White Beans with Tilapia

1 tablespoon whole wheat flour

1 tilapia fillet (4 ounces)

⅛ teaspoon salt

½ teaspoon Italian Spice Blend (page 86)

Pinch of ground black pepper

1½ teaspoons olive oil

½ cup sliced onion

2 cups chopped kale

½ cup canned no-salt-added white beans, rinsed and drained

1 teaspoon minced garlic

⅓ cup reduced-sodium chicken broth

1 teaspoon lemon juice

1. Spread the flour on a plate. Dredge the tilapia in the flour to coat evenly. Sprinkle the fish with the salt, spice blend, and pepper.

2. In a large skillet over medium-high heat, warm the oil. Cook the fish for 4 minutes, or until browned on one side. Flip, add the onion, and cook for 4 minutes, or until the fish is browned on the second side.

3. Remove the tilapia from the skillet and add the kale, beans, garlic, broth, and lemon juice. Cook until all of the liquid is gone and the kale and onion are tender.

4. Serve the tilapia next to the kale mixture.

PER SERVING: *295 calories, 18 g protein, 47 g carbohydrates, 7 g total fat, 1 g saturated fat, 10 g fiber, 374 mg sodium, 306 mg calcium, 1,355 mg potassium, 137 mg magnesium*

Dukkah-Spiced Pork Tenderloin with Broccoli and Quinoa

3 ounces pork tenderloin

1 tablespoon Dukkah spice mix (page 84)

1 teaspoon olive oil

1½ cups chopped broccoli

3 tablespoons fat-free plain yogurt

¼ teaspoon garlic powder

⅛ teaspoon salt

Ground black pepper

3 teaspoons lemon juice, divided

½ cup cooked quinoa, prepared according to the package directions

1. Preheat the oven to 350°F.

2. Coat the pork with the spice mix.

3. In a medium ovenproof skillet over medium-high heat, warm the oil. Cook the pork for 1 minute on each side. Place the skillet in the oven and cook the pork for 12 to 14 minutes, or until a thermometer inserted in the center reaches 145°F and the juices run clear.

4. Meanwhile, place a steamer basket in a large pot with a few inches of water. Bring to a boil over high heat. Steam the broccoli, covered, in the basket for 10 minutes, or until tender-crisp. Or place in a medium micro-waveable bowl with 2 to 3 tablespoons of water, cover, and microwave on high power for 3 to 4 minutes or until tender-crisp.

5. In a small bowl, combine the yogurt, garlic powder, salt, pepper to taste, and 1 teaspoon of the lemon juice. Pour over the cooked pork.

6. Top the broccoli with the remaining 2 teaspoons lemon juice and serve with the quinoa and pork.

PER SERVING: 359 calories, 30 g protein, 36 g carbohydrates, 12 g total fat, 2 g saturated fat, 8 g fiber, 498 mg sodium, 203 mg calcium, 1,129 mg potassium, 141 mg magnesium

Pork and Veggie Taco Salad Slaw

3 ounces pork tenderloin

3 teaspoons Tex-Mex Spice Blend (page 85), divided

¼ cup fat-free plain yogurt

1 teaspoon lemon juice

1 teaspoon olive oil

½ cup finely chopped broccoli

½ cup chopped red bell pepper

¼ cup canned no-salt-added white beans, rinsed and drained

1. Preheat the oven to 350°F.

2. Rub the pork with 2½ teaspoons of the spice blend. Place on a baking sheet and roast for 15 minutes, or until a thermometer inserted in the center reaches 145°F and the juices run clear. Let stand for 5 minutes and cut into ½" cubes.

3. Meanwhile, in a large bowl, whisk together the yogurt, lemon juice, olive oil, and the remaining ½ teaspoon spice blend. Add the cooked pork, broccoli, pepper, and beans amd mix well.

TIME-SAVING HINT: *This is a great way to use leftover pork tenderloin!*

PER SERVING: 298 calories, 29 g protein, 29 g carbohydrates, 8 g total fat, 1.5 g saturated fat, 7 g fiber, 290 mg sodium, 224 mg calcium, 1,197 mg potassium, 99 mg magnesium

White Bean and Kale Soup

1   teaspoon olive oil

1   teaspoon minced garlic

½   cup chopped onion

1   teaspoon Italian Spice Blend (page 86)

1½   cups reduced-sodium chicken broth

½   cup canned no-salt-added white beans, rinsed and drained

1   cup roughly chopped kale

Ground black pepper

1. In a medium saucepan over medium heat, warm the oil. Cook the garlic, onion, and spice blend for 3 minutes, or until the onion is translucent.

2. Add the broth and beans and bring to a boil. Reduce the heat to low and simmer for 5 minutes. Remove from the heat.

3. Puree the soup with a hand blender until smooth. Return to the stove top over medium-low heat. Stir in the kale. Cook for 5 minutes, or until the kale is soft. Add pepper to taste.

PER SERVING: 316 calories, 21 g protein, 46 g carbohydrates, 8 g total fat, 1.5 g saturated fat, 9 g fiber, 144 mg sodium, 234 mg calcium, 1,361 mg potassium, 111 mg magnesium

Tilapia with Kiwi-Avocado Salsa, Roasted Broccoli, and Quinoa

¼ cup fat-free plain yogurt

1 teaspoon Tex-Mex Spice Blend (page 85)

2 teaspoons lime juice, divided

1 tilapia fillet (4 ounces)

⅛ avocado, chopped

½ kiwifruit, chopped

1 tablespoon chopped onion

1 teaspoon finely chopped fresh cilantro or ¼ teaspoon dried

1 teaspoon finely chopped fresh flat-leaf parsley

Ground black pepper

1 cup broccoli, stems and florets sliced into bite-size pieces

1 teaspoon olive oil

½ cup cooked quinoa (prepared according to package directions)

1. Preheat the oven to 400°F. Line a baking sheet with foil.

2. In a small bowl, combine the yogurt, spice blend, and 1 teaspoon of the lime juice. Divide the marinade in half.

3. Brush half of the marinade on the tilapia, coating all sides evenly. Marinate for 10 minutes in a zip-top bag or a medium shallow bowl that is covered and refrigerated.

4. Meanwhile, in a small bowl, combine the avocado, kiwi, onion, cilantro, parsley, pepper to taste, and the remaining 1 teaspoon lime juice. Set aside.

5. In a medium bowl, toss the broccoli with the oil. Spread on the baking sheet and roast for 8 to 10 minutes, or until tender, or longer if you prefer broccoli softer. Remove from the oven and set aside on a plate.

6. Change the oven temperature to broil. Place the tilapia on the same baking sheet and cook for 2 minutes on each side, or until the fish flakes easily.

7. Serve the fish topped with the reserved avocado salsa. Top the quinoa and broccoli with the remaining yogurt sauce.

PER SERVING: 361 calories, 28 g protein, 38 g carbohydrates, 12 g total fat, 2 g saturated fat, 6 g fiber, 189 mg sodium, 204 mg calcium, 1,097 mg potassium, 131 mg magnesium

Red Bell Pepper Stuffed with Pork and Quinoa

1   large red bell pepper

3   ounces pork tenderloin

⅛   teaspoon ground black pepper + extra for seasoning

    Garlic powder

½   cup finely chopped broccoli

½   cup cooked quinoa (prepared according to package directions)

¼   cup fat-free plain yogurt

1   teaspoon minced garlic

⅛   teaspoon onion powder

⅛   teaspoon salt

1. Preheat the oven to 350°F.

2. Halve the bell pepper lengthwise, removing the seeds and membranes. Chop up one half and save the other for stuffing.

3. Season the pork with the black pepper and garlic powder to taste. Roast on a baking sheet for 10 minutes. Let cool slightly and cut into small pieces. (Leave the oven on.)

4. In a large bowl, combine the cooked pork, chopped bell pepper, broccoli, quinoa, yogurt, garlic, onion powder, salt, and ⅛ teaspoon black pepper.

5. Place the reserved bell pepper half on a baking sheet. Coat the outside and inside of the bell pepper with cooking spray. Fill with the pork mixture. Bake for 20 minutes, or until the bell pepper is soft and a thermometer inserted into the pork filling reaches 145°F.

TIME-SAVING HINT: *This is another great way to use leftover pork tenderloin and leftover quinoa!*

PER SERVING: 349 calories, 28 g protein, 37 g carbohydrates, 9 g total fat, 2 g saturated fat, 7 g fiber, 411 mg sodium, 175 mg calcium, 1,145 mg potassium, 123 mg magnesium

Massaged Kale Avocado Salad

1 cup finely chopped kale

1¼ teaspoons olive oil

⅛ teaspoon kosher salt

½ cup canned no-salt-added white beans, rinsed and drained

¼ avocado, cut into cubes

¼ cup chopped onion

¼ cup chopped red bell pepper

1 tablespoon lemon juice

1. Wash and dry your hands. In a large bowl, sprinkle the kale with the oil and salt. Massage the kale for 3 minutes, or until it begins to soften.

2. Wash your hands again. Add the beans, avocado, onion, bell pepper, and lemon juice and toss.

NOTE: *Massaged salads are a new trend in healthy eating. Massaging kale in olive oil and adding lemon juice helps break down some of the tough fibers in the leaves, making them easier to eat and digest while still getting all of the nutrition benefits. Chopping the leaves finely also helps kale's flavor shine without being overpowering, allowing the other ingredients to have equal playing time in each bite of salad. Unlike other massaged-salad recipes, this one calls for very little salt; the olive oil and lemon juice soften the kale leaves effectively!*

PER SERVING: 353 calories, 14 g protein, 45 g carbohydrates, 15 g total fat, 2 g saturated fat, 13 g fiber, 330 mg sodium, 215 mg calcium, 1,320 mg potassium, 122 mg magnesium

Success Story: David Oblas

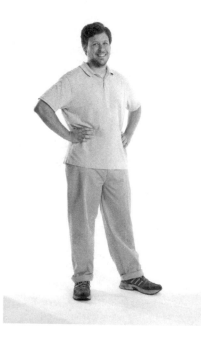

AGE: 28

HEIGHT: 6'

BLOOD PRESSURE IMPROVEMENT: David's systolic pressure fell 26 points, and his diastolic pressure dropped 16 points.

INCHES LOST: ¾" from his waist

"I was very hopeful that this would be a natural way to lower my blood pressure, and I was extremely pleased with the results," notes David. When he started the plan, his blood pressure was a high 145/89. Six weeks later, it was a healthy 119/73.

David and his wife, Kristi, went on the plan together and decided to keep on eating mineral-packed Power Foods from Phase 1 throughout the program. "They tasted great," he says. "I loved eating the peaches, kiwis, pork, and sweet potatoes. I enjoyed the spice mixes and was able to incorporate a lot of the fresh herbs from my garden. We're still eating a lot of peaches and kiwis, and we're constantly enjoying tilapia fillets. I'd never had quinoa, but I found it to be a pretty decent substitute for pasta, rice, and even breakfast grains, like oatmeal."

After the first week, the couple didn't want to leave these foods behind. "We were very happy to be able to expand our palates in Phase 2 but still kept the foods from Phase 1 prominent in our diets. We didn't really miss the salt so much. I think the moderate amount of sodium helped curb our cravings. Processed foods and restaurant foods definitely taste saltier to us!"

David took his blood pressure daily with a home monitor and saw the advantages of tracking this important health indicator. "I always made sure to take my blood pressure right when I woke up, and I took it again in the evening if I felt like I had a stressful day," he says. "I would say it helped me stay on track. I would always cheer when it was lower than the previous day. If it was higher, I would include more Power Mineral foods that day."

The good news? "I saw changes almost immediately," he says. "My blood pressure dropped quickly." He also saw drops in his blood pressure after doing the 5-minute meditation. "I didn't do it every day, but I would often meditate when I felt like I needed to relax," he says. "It definitely helped me get through some stressful days at work, and my blood pressure always went down afterward."

Doing the program together, he says, gave the couple a big advantage. They cooked together and motivated each other to exercise, too. Now, pairing up to pare down their blood pressure levels is still a perk. "Since the program ended, we have still been including many of the foods in our diets. All of the spice mixes are being used, and we're eating a lot of kale and broccoli, having tilapia at least once a week, and, in general, still incorporating all of the Phase 1 foods into our meals."

An unexpected bonus? "I can wear some old T-shirts that I own," he says. "My wife wasn't all that thrilled with my 'college' wardrobe, but I'm loving it."

CHAPTER 9

Phase 2: More Food, More Variety

Congratulations! You've finished Phase 1 of Lower Your Blood Pressure Naturally. You've spent the last week exploring and enjoying our 13 very special Power Foods. You've gotten a jump start on low-sodium, mineral-rich, calorie-controlled eating. And you may have already noticed changes in your weight and, if you monitor regularly, in your blood pressure. Many test panelists began seeing changes the first week.

Now the fun begins. In Phase 2—Weeks 2 through 6 of the plan—you'll eat a wider range of foods, have more meals (and more calories), and even have dessert several times a week. And we mean real dessert, like ice cream with a cookie, hot chocolate, peanut butter frozen yogurt, and more. In Phase 2, you'll continue to lose pounds and belly fat and to provide the mineral balance that reestablishes healthier blood pressure levels, thanks to less sodium and more calcium, potassium, and magnesium.

In Phase 2, you'll also have the freedom to eat out occasionally and to make lightning-fast meals at home using low-sodium frozen dinners paired with mineral-rich side dishes.

Phase 2 Eating

During Phase 2, you'll eat four meals plus a Power Mineral Smoothie or Power Mineral Dessert daily. For maximum mineral intake, be sure to choose at least one meal (breakfast, lunch, or dinner) daily from Phase 1 options in Chapter 8 along with three Phase 2 meals (again, any meal—breakfast, lunch, or dinner). And don't forget to treat yourself to a smoothie or a dessert daily. To get the most minerals, sip a smoothie 4 days a week and indulge in dessert 3 days a week.

A day of Phase 2 eating provides 1,500 to 1,550 calories, 2,300 milligrams of sodium or less, 1,200 milligrams of calcium, 420 milligrams of magnesium, and 4,700 milligrams of potassium. You also get all of the fiber, lean protein, good fats, and other nutrients—vitamins, minerals, and micronutrients—essential for great health.

We've provided a sample menu plan for a week of Phase 2 eating on page 132. Use the worksheets on pages 134–143 to map out your meals each week and the shopping list on pages 144–147 to make shopping each week a breeze.

Phase 2 Breakfasts

Breakfasts in Phase 2 provide around 350 calories along with at least 12 percent of the calcium and at least 20 percent of the magnesium and potassium you need daily. Each meal also contains less than 500 milligrams of sodium.

Apple-Cinnamon Muesli

⅓ cup rolled oats

⅛ teaspoon ground cinnamon + extra for sprinkling

1 tablespoon + 2 teaspoons chopped walnuts

½ cup fat-free milk

½ cup chopped apple

½ banana, sliced

¼ cup 0% plain Greek yogurt

1. In a small bowl, combine the oats, cinnamon, and walnuts. Pour the milk over the oat mixture and let sit for 5 minutes.

2. Top with the apple, banana, yogurt, and an extra sprinkle of cinnamon.

PER SERVING: 325 calories, 16 g protein, 52 g carbohydrates, 11 g total fat, 1 g saturated fat, 7 g fiber, 75 mg sodium, 252 mg calcium, 735 mg potassium, 98 mg magnesium

Blueberries and Cream Protein Pancakes

3 egg whites

⅓ cup rolled oats

⅛ teaspoon ground cinnamon

1 tablespoon sliced almonds

⅔ cup fat-free plain yogurt

⅔ cup blueberries

2 teaspoons maple syrup

1. In a medium bowl, whisk the egg whites with the oats, cinnamon, and almonds. Let sit for 5 minutes.

2. Heat a large skillet coated with cooking spray over medium-high heat. Pour half of the batter into the skillet and cook for 3 minutes, or until the pancake becomes firm. Flip and cook for 2 minutes, or until the remaining side is golden. Repeat with the other half of the batter.

3. Top the pancakes with the yogurt, blueberries, and maple syrup.

PER SERVING: 367 calories, 36 g protein, 56 g carbohydrates, 6 g total fat, 1 g saturated fat, 6 g fiber, 294 mg sodium, 379 mg calcium, 821 mg potassium, 103 mg magnesium

Open-Faced Avocado-Mozzarella Egg Sandwich

1 cup fresh spinach

1 egg

1 slice whole grain bread (see note)

2 tablespoons hummus

4 slices tomato

¼ avocado, sliced

1 ounce sliced reduced-fat mozzarella cheese

1. Preheat the broiler.

2. In a medium skillet coated with cooking spray over medium-high heat, cook the spinach, stirring frequently, for 30 seconds, or until just wilted. Transfer to a plate and set aside.

3. In a small skillet coated with cooking spray over medium-high heat, cook the egg your favorite way. Remove from the heat.

4. Toast the bread. Top with the hummus, tomato, avocado, reserved spinach, and cooked egg. Place the cheese on top.

5. Put the sandwich on a baking sheet or rack and broil for 2 minutes, or until the cheese is melted.

NOTE: *Look for bread with 160 mg of sodium or less per slice.*

PER SERVING: 355 calories, 21 g protein, 25 g carbohydrates, 21 g total fat, 7 g saturated fat, 8 g fiber, 419 mg sodium, 315 mg calcium, 790 mg potassium, 88 mg magnesium

Pear–Almond Butter Toast with Café au Lait

Toast

1 slice whole grain bread
(see note on opposite page)

1 tablespoon natural almond
butter

1 pear, sliced

Ground cinnamon

Café au Lait

1 cup fat-free milk

1 cup hot coffee

Ground cinnamon

1. *To make the toast:* Toast the bread. Spread the almond butter on the toast and top with the pear slices. Sprinkle with the cinnamon to taste.

2. *To make the café au lait:* In a large microwaveable mug, heat the milk in the microwave on high power for 45 seconds. Add the coffee. Or in a small saucepan over medium heat, warm the milk for 2 minutes, or until steaming. Place the coffee in a large mug and add the warmed milk. Sprinkle with the cinnamon to taste.

PER SERVING: 363 calories, 15 g protein, 55 g carbohydrates, 11 g total fat, 1 g saturated fat, 8 g fiber, 300 mg sodium, 390 mg calcium, 791 mg potassium, 113 mg magnesium

Black Bean Breakfast Tostadas

1 egg + 1 egg white

1 teaspoon olive oil

1 ½ cups fresh baby spinach

½ cup canned no-salt-added black beans, rinsed and drained

2 corn tortillas (6" diameter)

4 tablespoons 0% plain Greek yogurt

2 tablespoons salsa

1. In a small bowl, whisk the eggs.

2. In a medium skillet over medium-high heat, warm the oil. Cook the eggs and spinach, stirring occasionally, for 3 to 4 minutes, or until the eggs are set and the spinach is wilted. Remove from the heat.

3. In a small saucepan over medium heat, warm the beans for 3 to 4 minutes or until heated through.

4. Top each tortilla with half of the beans, egg mixture, yogurt, and salsa.

PER SERVING: 356 calories, 28 g protein, 47 g carbohydrates, 7 g total fat, 2 g saturated fat, 12 g fiber, 337 mg sodium, 203 mg calcium, 896 mg potassium, 149 mg magnesium

Cheesy Potato Hash Topped with an Egg

1½ teaspoons olive oil

¾ cup finely chopped potato

½ cup chopped onion

1½ cups fresh baby spinach

Ground black pepper

⅛ teaspoon kosher salt or sea salt

¼ cup (1 ounce) shredded reduced-fat Cheddar cheese

1 egg

½ cup finely chopped tomato

1. In a large skillet over medium heat, warm the oil. Cook the potato and onion, stirring occasionally, for 8 to 10 minutes, or until the potato is browned on the outside and soft inside. Add the spinach and cook for 1 minute, or until just wilted. Sprinkle with the pepper to taste and the salt. Stir in the cheese and remove from heat.

2. In a small skillet coated with cooking spray over medium-high heat, cook the egg your favorite way.

3. Serve the egg over the hash. Top with the tomato.

PER SERVING: 358 calories, 19 g protein, 34 g carbohydrates, 17 g total fat, 6 g saturated fat, 5 g fiber, 325 mg sodium, 370 mg calcium, 1,146 mg potassium, 95 mg magnesium

French Toast with Bananas and Almonds

1 egg

¼ cup fat-free milk

½ teaspoon vanilla extract

2 slices whole wheat bread
   (see note on page 108)

¾ banana, sliced

2 tablespoons 0% plain Greek
   yogurt

1 tablespoon sliced almonds

1. In a shallow bowl large enough for a slice of bread to lay flat, whisk together the egg, milk, and vanilla.

2. Heat a medium skillet coated with cooking spray over medium heat. Dip the bread into the egg mixture and cook for 2 to 3 minutes on each side, or until both sides are browned and slightly crispy.

3. Top with the banana, yogurt, and almonds.

PER SERVING: *375 calories, 22 g protein, 52 g carbohydrates, 10 g total fat, 2 g saturated fat, 8 g fiber, 354 mg sodium, 219 mg calcium, 726 mg potassium, 105 mg magnesium*

Phase 2 Lunches and Dinners

Phase 2 lunches and dinners also provide an average of 350 calories as well as at least 12 percent of your daily calcium and at least 20 percent of your daily magnesium and potassium. Each meal also contains less than 500 milligrams of sodium.

Veggie and Cheddar Frittata

2   eggs + 2 egg whites

1   tablespoon water

¼   teaspoon Italian Spice Blend (page 86)

1   teaspoon olive oil

⅓   cup chopped onion

⅓   cup finely chopped mushrooms

3   cups fresh spinach

¼   cup (1 ounce) shredded reduced-fat Cheddar cheese

1. Preheat the broiler.

2. In a small bowl, whisk together the eggs, water, and spice blend. Set aside.

3. In a small ovenproof skillet over medium-high heat, warm the oil. Cook the onion and mushrooms for 4 minutes, or until soft and golden. Add the spinach and cook for 2 minutes.

4. Pour the reserved egg mixture over the veggies, sprinkle with the cheese, and cook for 3 to 4 minutes, or until the eggs begin to set.

5. Transfer the skillet to the oven and broil for 3 to 4 minutes, or until the eggs are set and the top is golden.

PER SERVING: 341 calories, 31 g protein, 11 g carbohydrates, 20 g total fat, 7 g saturated fat, 3 g fiber, 529 mg sodium, 415 mg calcium, 921 mg potassium, 108 mg magnesium

Fiesta Shrimp Tacos

1 teaspoon olive oil

¼ pound (4 ounces) large shrimp, peeled and deveined

¾ cup shredded cabbage

⅓ cup shredded carrot

⅓ cup fat-free plain yogurt

2 corn tortillas (6" diameter)

2 tablespoons salsa

2 tablespoons chopped avocado

1. In a medium skillet over medium-high heat, warm the oil. Cook the shrimp for 2 minutes on each side, or until opaque. Remove from the heat.

2. In a medium bowl, toss the cabbage and carrot with the yogurt.

3. Divide the cabbage mixture evenly between the tortillas. Top each with half of the shrimp, salsa, and avocado.

PER SERVING: 355 calories, 32 g protein, 38 g carbohydrates, 10 g total fat, 1.5 g saturated fat, 7 g fiber, 435 mg sodium, 312 mg calcium, 969 mg potassium, 111 mg magnesium

Orange-Ginger Halibut

½ cup reduced-sodium chicken broth

½ cup water

1 teaspoon finely chopped fresh ginger

½ cup orange juice

¼ teaspoon reduced-sodium soy sauce

4 ounces halibut

3 cups fresh spinach

1 cup cooked bulgur (prepared according to package directions)

1 teaspoon olive oil

2 teaspoons sliced almonds

Pinch of ground black pepper

1. In a medium skillet over medium-high heat, bring the broth, water, ginger, orange juice, and soy sauce to a simmer.

2. Add the halibut, cover, and cook for 4 minutes on each side, or until the fish is opaque.

3. Remove the fish and set aside. Boil the remaining liquid for 5 minutes, or until it's reduced by half.

4. Add the spinach and cook for 2 minutes, or until just wilted. Remove from the heat.

5. Toss the bulgur with the oil, almonds, and pepper. Arrange in the center of a plate. Top with the spinach and reserved halibut.

PER SERVING: 347 calories, 31 g protein, 38 g carbohydrates, 9 g total fat, 1 g saturated fat, 7 g fiber, 202 mg sodium, 149 mg calcium, 1,368 mg potassium, 165 mg magnesium

Garlic-Ginger Tofu Stir-Fry

2 teaspoons olive oil, divided

¼ block tofu, drained and chopped into ½" cubes

2 teaspoons minced garlic, divided

½ cup shredded cabbage

2 cups sliced baby bok choy

¼ cup sliced onion

¼ cup sliced mushrooms

2 tablespoons reduced-sodium chicken broth

1 teaspoon finely chopped fresh ginger

½ teaspoon reduced-sodium soy sauce

1 cup cooked bulgur (prepared according to package directions)

1. In a large skillet over medium-high heat, warm 1 teaspoon of the oil. Cook the tofu and 1 teaspoon of the garlic, stirring every 30 seconds, for 8 minutes, or until the tofu is browned on the sides. Remove the tofu mixture and set aside in a bowl.

2. In the same skillet, warm the remaining 1 teaspoon oil. Cook the cabbage, bok choy, onion, and mushrooms, stirring every minute, for 4 minutes, or until soft and golden.

3. Add the tofu back to the skillet and stir in the broth, ginger, soy sauce, and the remaining 1 teaspoon garlic (if you love garlic!). Cook for 1 minute, stirring to combine.

4. Serve over the bulgur.

PER SERVING: 337 calories, 18 g protein, 39 g carbohydrates, 15 g total fat, 2 g saturated fat, 10 g fiber, 203 mg sodium, 362 mg calcium, 823 mg potassium, 133 mg magnesium

Open-Faced Tuna Melt

½ can (2.5 ounces) water-packed tuna, drained

1½ tablespoons 0% plain Greek yogurt

Pinch of ground black pepper

2 tablespoons finely chopped onion

3 slices tomato

1 slice whole grain bread (see note on page 108)

1½ ounces sliced Cheddar cheese

½ cup cucumber slices

1 banana

1. Preheat the broiler.

2. In a small bowl, mix together the tuna, yogurt, pepper, and onion.

3. Place the tomato slices on the bread and top with the tuna mixture and cheese. Place on a baking sheet and broil for 3 minutes, or until the cheese is melted.

4. Serve with the cucumber and banana.

PER SERVING: 367 calories, 38 g protein, 35 g carbohydrates, 9 g total fat, 5 g saturated fat, 5 g fiber, 606 mg sodium, 451 mg calcium, 1,023 mg potassium, 95 mg magnesium

Chopped Chicken Salad

1 cup shredded cabbage

½ cup shredded carrot

3 ounces cooked chicken breast, chopped

⅓ cup no-salt-added kidney beans, rinsed and drained

¼ cup fat-free plain yogurt

2 teaspoons lemon juice

½ teaspoon minced garlic

2 teaspoons Dukkah spice blend (page 84)

1 tablespoon sliced almonds

1. In a medium bowl, toss together the cabbage, carrot, chicken, and beans.

2. In a small bowl, whisk together the yogurt, lemon juice, garlic, and spice blend. Stir into the chicken mixture. Sprinkle with the almonds.

PER SERVING: 360 calories, 39 g protein, 31 g carbohydrates, 9 g total fat, 1 g saturated fat, 9 g fiber, 295 mg sodium, 230 mg calcium, 1,262 mg potassium, 114 mg magnesium

Yogurt-Marinated Chicken with Baked Potato and Swiss Chard

½ cup 0% plain Greek yogurt

1 teaspoon lemon juice

1 teaspoon Indian Spice Blend (page 85)

1 teaspoon minced garlic, divided

1 boneless, skinless chicken thigh (3 ounces)

1 small potato

1 teaspoon olive oil

2 cups roughly chopped Swiss chard

1. Coat a grill rack or grill pan with cooking spray, or if baking, lightly coat a baking pan with cooking spray. Preheat the grill, or preheat the oven to 400°F.

2. In a small bowl, combine the yogurt, lemon juice, spice blend, and ½ teaspoon of the garlic.

3. In a medium bowl, top the chicken with half of the yogurt mixture. Turn the chicken to coat and marinate for 15 minutes.

4. Meanwhile, poke a few holes in the potato and microwave on high power for 4 minutes, or until cooked through.

5. In a medium skillet over medium heat, warm the oil. Cook the Swiss chard and the remaining ½ teaspoon garlic for 5 minutes, or until the chard is wilted. Remove from the heat.

6. On a grill or in a grill pan heated over medium-high heat on the stove top, cook the chicken for 4 to 5 minutes on each side, or until a thermometer inserted in the thickest portion registers 165°F and the juices run clear. If using the oven, bake for 20 minutes, or until a thermometer inserted in the thickest portion registers 165°F and the juices run clear.

7. Top the potato with the remaining yogurt mixture. Serve with the chard and chicken.

PER SERVING: 356 calories, 33 g protein, 37 g carbohydrates, 9 g total fat, 2 g saturated fat, 429 mg sodium, 5 g fiber, 206 mg calcium, 1,471 mg potassium, 134 mg magnesium

Corn Tortilla Pizzas

2 corn tortillas (6" diameter)

1 teaspoon olive oil

2 cups fresh baby spinach

½ cup shredded reduced-fat mozzarella cheese

1 cup chopped tomato

1 teaspoon Italian Spice Blend (page 86)

1. Preheat the oven or toaster oven to 400°F. Line a baking sheet or toaster oven tray with foil.

2. Coat the tortillas with cooking spray on both sides and place on the baking sheet or tray.

3. In a medium skillet over medium-high heat, warm the oil. Cook the spinach for 2 minutes, or until just wilted.

4. Divide the cheese, tomato, and cooked spinach evenly between the tortillas. Sprinkle with the spice blend (add more if you like). Bake for 8 to 10 minutes, or until the tortillas are crispy and the cheese is melted.

PER SERVING: 361 calories, 21 g protein, 33 g carbohydrates, 18 g total fat, 8 g saturated fat, 7 g fiber, 376 mg sodium, 529 mg calcium, 904 mg potassium, 116 mg magnesium

BBQ Shrimp and Veggie Kebabs with Cheddar Parsnip Mash

¼ pound large shrimp, peeled and deveined

3 teaspoons olive oil, divided

1 teaspoon BBQ Rub (page 86)

⅓ cup grape tomatoes

⅓ cup quartered mushrooms

⅓ cup onion wedges

½ parsnip, peeled and quartered

2 tablespoons fat-free milk

1 tablespoon 0% plain Greek yogurt

¼ cup (1 ounce) shredded reduced-fat Cheddar cheese

⅛ teaspoon salt

Ground black pepper

1. On a wooden or metal skewer, thread the shrimp. Brush with 1 teaspoon of the oil and sprinkle with the rub, covering both sides of the shrimp. Set aside on a plate.

2. On another skewer, alternately thread the tomatoes, mushrooms, and onion. Brush the vegetables with 1 teaspoon of the oil and set aside on the plate with the shrimp.

3. In a medium saucepan, add the parsnip and cover with water. Bring to a boil over high heat. Reduce the heat to low, cover, and simmer for 15 minutes, or until tender. Drain and set the parsnip aside.

4. Meanwhile, coat a grill rack with cooking spray. Preheat the grill to medium.

5. Return the saucepan to the heat. Add the milk, yogurt, and the remaining 1 teaspoon oil and mix well. Add the reserved parsnip and mash, leaving small chunks for texture. Stir in the cheese, salt, and pepper to taste. Cover and remove from the heat.

6. Grill the reserved shrimp and veggie kebabs until the shrimp are opaque and the veggies are tender, about 5 minutes for the shrimp and 10 minutes for the veggies. Serve with the mashed parsnip.

PER SERVING: 369 calories, 32 g protein, 25 g carbohydrates, 17 g total fat, 6 g saturated fat, 5 g fiber, 280 mg sodium, 309 mg calcium, 977 mg potassium, 88 mg magnesium

Tex-Mex Black Bean and Bulgur Burger

1   egg

⅓   cup no-salt-added black beans, rinsed and drained

¼   cup cooked bulgur (prepared according to package directions)

⅓   cup chopped mushrooms

1   tablespoon chopped fresh flat-leaf parsley

1   teaspoon Tex-Mex Spice Blend (page 85)

2   teaspoons olive oil, divided

2   thick slices onion

1   cup broccoli, chopped and lightly steamed

¼   cup (1 ounce) shredded reduced-fat Cheddar cheese

2   tablespoons salsa

1. In a small bowl, whisk the egg. (You'll use just half of it in this recipe.)

2. In a medium bowl, mash the beans. Add the bulgur, mushrooms, parsley, spice blend, and half of the egg and mix well. Form the mixture into a patty.

3. In a small skillet over medium-high heat, warm 1 teaspoon of the oil. Add the patty and onion. Cook the patty for 3 minutes on each side, or until heated through and lightly crisped on the outside. Remove from the heat.

4. Toss the broccoli with the remaining 1 teaspoon oil.

5. Top the patty with the cheese, cooked onion, and salsa. Serve with the broccoli.

NOTE: *This recipe calls for using just half of an egg to meet calorie guidelines. Why not double this recipe? You'll use the whole egg and have an extra burger for tomorrow!*

PER SERVING: 355 calories, 21 g protein, 32 g carbohydrates, 18 g total fat, 5.5 g saturated fat, 9 g fiber, 472 mg sodium, 350 mg calcium, 739 mg potassium, 100 mg magnesium

Garlic-Lime Tofu Sandwich with Hummus, Avocado, and Tomato

1 tablespoon lime juice

1 teaspoon minced garlic

½ teaspoon chili powder

⅛ teaspoon kosher salt

⅛ teaspoon ground red pepper

⅕ block extra-firm tofu, drained and cut into ½" slices

1 teaspoon olive oil

2 slices whole wheat bread (see note on page 108)

1 tablespoon hummus

⅛ avocado, sliced

2 slices tomato

¼ cup cucumber slices

½ cup fresh baby spinach

1. In a medium bowl, mix together the lime juice, garlic, chili powder, salt, and pepper. Add the tofu, toss to coat, and marinate for 5 to 10 minutes.

2. In a large skillet over medium-high heat, warm the oil. Cook the tofu for 3 minutes on each side, or until browned.

3. Toast the bread. Spread the hummus on 1 slice and add the tofu, avocado, tomato, cucumber, and spinach. Top with the other slice of bread. Cut the sandwich in half and enjoy.

PER SERVING: 366 calories, 20 g protein, 37 g carbohydrates, 17 g total fat, 2 g saturated fat, 9 g fiber, 324 mg sodium, 273 mg calcium, 726 mg potassium, 138 mg magnesium

Power Mineral Smoothies and Desserts

Choose a smoothie or a dessert every day during Phase 2. For optimal nutrition, we recommend alternating between the two so that you have smoothies four times a week and desserts three times a week.

Each smoothie contains around 200 calories and provides at least 35 percent of the calcium and at least 15 percent of the magnesium and potassium you need daily. Each dessert also has about 200 calories along with at least 15 percent of the calcium and at least 5 percent of the magnesium and potassium you need every day for good blood pressure control.

Tropical Greens Smoothie

1   cup unsweetened soy milk or fat-free milk

½   banana, cut into chunks and frozen

½   cup pineapple chunks (fresh, frozen, or canned in their own juice and drained)

1   cup fresh baby spinach

2   teaspoons unsweetened coconut flakes

Ice (optional)

In a blender, combine the soy milk, banana, pineapple, spinach, and coconut. Blend until smooth. Add the ice as needed for a frothier smoothie.

PER SERVING: 210 calories, 9 g protein, 30 g carbohydrates, 8 g total fat, 3 g saturated fat, 5 g fiber, 112 mg sodium, 343 mg calcium, 788 mg potassium, 92 mg magnesium

Chocolate-Nut Butter Banana Smoothie

¼ cup unsweetened soy milk or fat-free milk

½ cup fat-free plain yogurt

½ banana, cut into chunks and frozen

2 teaspoons natural almond butter or peanut butter

2 teaspoons unsweetened cocoa powder

Ice (optional)

In a blender, combine the milk, yogurt, banana, nut butter, and cocoa powder. Blend until smooth. Add the ice as needed for a frothier smoothie.

PER SERVING: 215 calories, 12 g protein, 28 g carbohydrates, 8 g total fat, 1 g saturated fat, 4 g fiber, 118 mg sodium, 363 mg calcium, 733 mg potassium, 97 mg magnesium

Orange-Carrot Creamsicle Smoothie

¾ cup fat-free plain yogurt

⅔ cup orange juice

½ cup shredded carrot

½ cup ice

In a blender, combine the yogurt, orange juice, carrot, and ice. Blend until smooth. Add more ice if needed to achieve the desired consistency.

PER SERVING: 207 calories, 12 g protein, 39 g carbohydrates, 1 g total fat, 0 g saturated fat, 2 g fiber, 183 mg sodium, 402 mg calcium, 940 mg potassium, 60 mg magnesium

Berries and Cream Smoothie

¾ cup fat-free plain yogurt

¼ cup fat-free milk or
   unsweetened soy milk

½ cup frozen blueberries

5 fresh or frozen strawberries,
   stems removed

1 teaspoon honey

   Ice (optional)

In a blender, combine the yogurt, milk, blueberries, strawberries, and honey. Blend until smooth. Add the ice as needed for a frothier smoothie.

PER SERVING: 206 calories, 14 g protein, 38 g carbohydrates, 1 g total fat, 0 g saturated fat, 3 g fiber, 169 mg sodium, 455 mg calcium, 717 mg potassium, 54 mg magnesium

Pear-Ginger-Kale Smoothie

½ cup fat-free plain yogurt

½ cup fat-free milk or
   unsweetened soy milk

½ small apple

½ small pear

½ cup roughly chopped kale

1 teaspoon grated fresh ginger

   Ice (optional)

In a blender, combine the yogurt, milk, apple, pear, kale, and ginger. Blend until smooth. Add the ice as needed for a frothier smoothie.

PER SERVING: 209 calories, 13 g protein, 40 g carbohydrates, 1 g total fat, 0 g saturated fat, 5 g fiber, 160 mg sodium, 455 mg calcium, 842 mg potassium, 62 mg magnesium

Peach-Almond Ice Cream Cup

½ cup light vanilla ice cream (such as Breyers or Edy's Slow Churned)

½ cup peach slices (fresh, frozen and thawed, or canned in their own juice and drained)

2 tablespoons sliced almonds

In a small bowl, top the ice cream with the peach slices and almonds. Enjoy!

PER SERVING: 209 calories, 7 g protein, 27 g carbohydrates, 9 g total fat, 2 g saturated fat, 3 g fiber, 48 mg sodium, 151 mg calcium, 230 mg potassium, 39 mg magnesium

Make-Ahead Maple-Walnut Chia Pudding

Letting the ingredients "marinate" in the refrigerator for at least 8 hours makes the chia seeds swell and soften to become a pudding. Make it tonight to enjoy tomorrow, or toss together in the morning for an after-dinner treat.

½ cup unsweetened soy milk or fat-free milk

¼ cup banana slices, mashed

1 tablespoon chia seeds

2 teaspoons maple syrup

½ teaspoon vanilla extract

¼ teaspoon ground cinnamon

1 tablespoon chopped walnuts

1. In a small bowl, whisk the milk, banana, chia seeds, maple syrup, vanilla, and cinnamon for 1 minute, or until blended well.

2. Cover tightly with plastic wrap and refrigerate for 8 hours or overnight.

3. When ready to eat, top with the walnuts.

PER SERVING: 215 calories, 7 g protein, 22 g carbohydrates, 11 g total fat, 1 g saturated fat, 7 g fiber, 46 mg sodium, 255 mg calcium, 392 mg potassium, 91 mg magnesium

Double-Dark Hot Chocolate

1¼ cups vanilla soy milk or fat-free milk + 1 teaspoon vanilla extract

2 teaspoons unsweetened cocoa powder

1 teaspoon sugar

Pinch of ground cinnamon (optional)

1 tablespoon dark chocolate chips

1. In a small saucepan over medium heat, warm the milk for 5 minutes, or until steaming.

2. Add the cocoa powder, sugar, and cinnamon (if desired) and cook, stirring constantly, for 3 minutes, or until well combined.

3. Add the chocolate and cook, stirring constantly, for 1 minute, or until the chocolate is melted.

Microwave directions: In a large microwaveable cup, stir together the milk, cocoa powder, sugar, and cinnamon (if desired). Microwave on high power for 30 seconds and stir. Add the chocolate and microwave for 1 minute, or until the chocolate is melted and the milk is steaming.

PER SERVING: 189 calories, 9 g protein, 24 g carbohydrates, 8 g total fat, 2.5 g saturated fat, 3 g fiber, 121 mg sodium, 380 mg calcium, 452 mg potassium, 76 mg magnesium

Peanut Butter–Banana Frozen Yogurt

½ cup low-fat vanilla yogurt, divided among ice cube tray sections and frozen

½ banana, cut into chunks and frozen

2 teaspoons natural peanut butter

Ground cinnamon (optional)

1. In a blender or food processor, combine the yogurt cubes and banana. Blend or process on high, scraping down the sides every minute, for 3 minutes, or until the mixture holds together.

2. Add the peanut butter and blend on high for 30 seconds, or until the mixture is creamy, like soft-serve ice cream.

3. Serve immediately, sprinkled with the cinnamon to taste (if desired).

PER SERVING: 211 calories, 9 g protein, 31 g carbohydrates, 7 g total fat, 2 g saturated fat, 2 g fiber, 130 mg sodium, 217 mg calcium, 518 mg potassium, 50 mg magnesium

Kiwi-Ginger Ice Cream Cookie Cup

½ cup light vanilla ice cream (such as Breyers or Edy's Slow Churned)

1 kiwifruit, peeled and chopped

1 small gingersnap cookie

½ tablespoon sliced almonds

1. In a medium bowl, let the ice cream soften for 5 to 10 minutes, or until it's easy to stir but not runny. Stir in the kiwi.

2. Place the gingersnap into the bottom of a cupcake paper. Top with the ice cream mixture. Sprinkle with the almonds.

3. Put in the freezer in a sealed container until ready to eat.

PER SERVING: 202 calories, 5 g protein, 34 g carbohydrates, 6 g total fat, 2 g saturated fat, 3 g fiber, 96 mg sodium, 154 mg calcium, 282 mg potassium, 96 mg magnesium

Fast, Easy Lunches

Egg Salad Sandwich with Swiss, Spinach, and Tomato

1 hard-cooked egg and 1 hard-cooked egg white, chopped

1 tablespoon 0% plain Greek yogurt

1 teaspoon light mayonnaise

2 tablespoons chopped celery

2 tablespoons chopped onion

Ground black pepper

Garlic powder

¾ ounce sliced Swiss cheese

½ cup fresh baby spinach

2 slices tomato

2 slices whole grain bread (see note on page 108)

In a small bowl, combine the eggs, yogurt, mayo, celery, and onion. Add the pepper and garlic powder to taste. Place the egg salad, cheese, spinach, and tomato between the slices of bread.

PER SERVING: 375 calories, 27 g protein, 31 g carbohydrates, 16 g total fat, 7 g saturated fat, 471 mg sodium, 5 g fiber, 359 mg calcium, 546 mg potassium, 88 mg magnesium

Chicken Sandwich with Roasted Peppers, Spinach, and Provolone

1 tablespoon hummus

2 slices whole grain bread (see note on page 108)

3 ounces skinless roasted chicken breast

½ cup sliced roasted red bell peppers

½ cup fresh baby spinach

½ ounce sliced reduced-fat provolone cheese

Spread the hummus on 1 slice of bread. Add the chicken, peppers, spinach, and cheese. Top with the other slice of bread.

PER SERVING: 358 calories, 39 g protein, 29 g carbohydrates, 9 g total fat, 3 g saturated fat, 460 mg sodium, 5 g fiber, 206 mg calcium, 534 mg potassium, 95 mg magnesium

Avocado, Provolone, Hummus, Cucumber, and Tomato Sandwich

1½ tablespoons hummus

2 slices whole grain bread (see note on page 108)

¾ ounce sliced reduced-fat provolone cheese

¼ cup sliced cucumber

2 slices tomato

¼ avocado, sliced

Spread the hummus on 1 slice of bread. Add the cheese, cucumber, tomato, and avocado. Top with the other slice of bread.

PER SERVING: 346 calories, 17 g protein, 35 g carbohydrates, 16 g total fat, 5 g saturated fat, 530 mg sodium, 9 g fiber, 297 mg calcium, 593 mg potassium, 83 mg magnesium

Salad Bar Lunch

2 cups mixed greens

½ cup chopped tomato

½ cup sliced cucumber

¼ cup chickpeas (or kidney, black, or white beans)

2 ounces chicken breast

2 tablespoons feta cheese

1 tablespoon sunflower seeds

1 tablespoon vinegar (any type)

1 teaspoon olive oil

In a large bowl, add the greens, tomato, cucumber, chickpeas or beans, chicken, cheese, and sunflower seeds. Dress with the vinegar and oil.

PER SERVING: 352 calories, 28 g protein, 26 g carbohydrates, 16 g total fat, 5 g saturated fat, 413 mg sodium, 6 g fiber, 214 mg calcium, 1,082 mg potassium, 93 mg magnesium

Phase 2 Menu Planning

Wondering what a day—or a whole week—of Phase 2 eating will look and taste like? Here's a sample menu plan, followed by five pages of worksheets for planning your own weekly menus.

Reminder: Each day, choose one meal from Phase 1, three from Phase 2, and a Power Mineral Smoothie or Power Mineral Dessert. Use your fourth meal as a hearty snack or combine two meals to make a large meal to enjoy for breakfast, lunch, or dinner. Aim to have a smoothie four times a week and a dessert three times a week to get the most minerals.

Monday

BREAKFAST: Peaches and Cream Hot Quinoa Cereal, page 87 (Phase 1 meal)

LUNCH: Open-Faced Avocado-Mozzarella Egg Sandwich, page 108

AFTERNOON SNACK: Pear–Almond Butter Toast with Café au Lait, page 109

DINNER: BBQ Shrimp and Veggie Kebabs with Cheddar Parsnip Mash, page 121 (make extra for tomorrow)

DESSERT: Double-Dark Hot Chocolate, page 128

Tuesday

BREAKFAST: Black Bean Breakfast Tostadas, page 110

LUNCH: Massaged Kale Avocado Salad, page 101 (Phase 1 Meal)

AFTERNOON SNACK: BBQ Shrimp and Veggie Kebabs with Cheddar Parsnip Mash (leftovers from Monday)

DINNER: Corn Tortilla Pizzas, page 120 (make extra for tomorrow)

SMOOTHIE: Tropical Greens Smoothie, page 124

Wednesday

BREAKFAST: Kiwi-Peach Yogurt Parfait, page 88 (Phase 1 meal)

LUNCH: Garlic-Lime Tofu Sandwich with Hummus, Avocado, and Tomato, page 123

AFTERNOON SNACK: Corn Tortilla Pizzas (leftovers from Tuesday)

DINNER: Fiesta Shrimp Tacos, page 114

DESSERT: Peanut Butter–Banana Frozen Yogurt, page 129

Thursday

BREAKFAST: Blueberries and Cream Protein Pancakes, page 107

MORNING SNACK: Apple-Cinnamon Muesli, page 106

LUNCH: Avocado, Provolone, Hummus, Cucumber, and Tomato Sandwich, page 131

DINNER: Twice-Baked Spiced Sweet Potato with Roasted Broccoli and Tilapia, page 91 (Phase 1 meal)

SMOOTHIE: Chocolate–Nut Butter Banana Smoothie, page 125

Friday

BREAKFAST: Open-Faced Avocado-Mozzarella Egg Sandwich, page 108

LUNCH: Kale Salad with Roasted Peaches, Spiced Yogurt-Avocado Dressing, and Tilapia, page 93 (Phase 1 meal)

AFTERNOON SNACK: Pear–Almond Butter Toast with Café au Lait, page 109

DINNER: Fiesta Shrimp Tacos, page 114

SMOOTHIE: Orange-Carrot Creamsicle Smoothie, page 125

Saturday

BREAKFAST: Peaches and Cream Hot Quinoa Cereal, page 87 (Phase 1 meal)

LUNCH: Open-Faced Tuna Melt, page 117

AFTERNOON SNACK: French Toast with Bananas and Almonds, page 112

DINNER: Chopped Chicken Salad, page 118 (make extra for tomorrow)

SMOOTHIE: Pear-Ginger-Kale Smoothie, page 126

Sunday

BREAKFAST: French Toast with Bananas and Almonds, page 112

LUNCH: White Bean–Sweet Potato Patties over Kale Topped with Yogurt Sauce, page 94 (Phase 1 meal)

AFTERNOON SNACK: Chopped Chicken Salad (leftovers from Saturday)

DINNER: Pork Stir-Fry with Quinoa, page 92 (Phase 1 meal)

DESSERT: Peach-Almond Ice Cream Cup, page 127

Menu Planning Worksheets

Phase 2: Week 2 of Lower Your Blood Pressure Naturally

Monday

BREAKFAST: _____

LUNCH: _____

DINNER: _____

SMOOTHIE OR DESSERT: _____

SNACK: _____

Tuesday

BREAKFAST: _____

LUNCH: _____

DINNER: _____

SMOOTHIE OR DESSERT: _____

SNACK: _____

Wednesday

BREAKFAST: _____

LUNCH: _____

DINNER: _____

SMOOTHIE OR DESSERT: _____

SNACK: _____

Thursday

BREAKFAST: _____

LUNCH: _____

DINNER: _____

SMOOTHIE OR DESSERT: _____

SNACK: _____

Friday

BREAKFAST: _____

LUNCH: _____

DINNER: _____

SMOOTHIE OR DESSERT: _____

SNACK: _____

Saturday

BREAKFAST: _____

LUNCH: _____

DINNER: _____

SMOOTHIE OR DESSERT: _____

SNACK: _____

Sunday

BREAKFAST: _____

LUNCH: _____

DINNER: _____

SMOOTHIE OR DESSERT: _____

SNACK: _____

Menu Planning Worksheet

Phase 2: Week 3 of Lower Your Blood Pressure Naturally

Monday
BREAKFAST: _____
LUNCH: _____
DINNER: _____
SMOOTHIE OR DESSERT: _____
SNACK: _____

Tuesday
BREAKFAST: _____
LUNCH: _____
DINNER: _____
SMOOTHIE OR DESSERT: _____
SNACK: _____

Wednesday
BREAKFAST: _____
LUNCH: _____
DINNER: _____
SMOOTHIE OR DESSERT: _____
SNACK: _____

Thursday
BREAKFAST: _____
LUNCH: _____
DINNER: _____
SMOOTHIE OR DESSERT: _____
SNACK: _____

Friday

BREAKFAST: _____

LUNCH: _____

DINNER: _____

SMOOTHIE OR DESSERT: _____

SNACK: _____

Saturday

BREAKFAST: _____

LUNCH: _____

DINNER: _____

SMOOTHIE OR DESSERT: _____

SNACK: _____

Sunday

BREAKFAST: _____

LUNCH: _____

DINNER: _____

SMOOTHIE OR DESSERT: _____

SNACK: _____

Menu Planning Worksheet

Phase 2: Week 4 of Lower Your Blood Pressure Naturally

Monday

BREAKFAST: _____

LUNCH: _____

DINNER: _____

SMOOTHIE OR DESSERT: _____

SNACK: _____

Tuesday

BREAKFAST: _____

LUNCH: _____

DINNER: _____

SMOOTHIE OR DESSERT: _____

SNACK: _____

Wednesday

BREAKFAST: _____

LUNCH: _____

DINNER: _____

SMOOTHIE OR DESSERT: _____

SNACK: _____

Thursday

BREAKFAST: _____

LUNCH: _____

DINNER: _____

SMOOTHIE OR DESSERT: _____

SNACK: _____

Friday

BREAKFAST: _____

LUNCH: _____

DINNER: _____

SMOOTHIE OR DESSERT: _____

SNACK: _____

Saturday

BREAKFAST: _____

LUNCH: _____

DINNER: _____

SMOOTHIE OR DESSERT: _____

SNACK: _____

Sunday

BREAKFAST: _____

LUNCH: _____

DINNER: _____

SMOOTHIE OR DESSERT: _____

SNACK: _____

Menu Planning Worksheet

Phase 2: Week 5 of Lower Your Blood Pressure Naturally

Monday

BREAKFAST: _____

LUNCH: _____

DINNER: _____

SMOOTHIE OR DESSERT: _____

SNACK: _____

Tuesday

BREAKFAST: _____

LUNCH: _____

DINNER: _____

SMOOTHIE OR DESSERT: _____

SNACK: _____

Wednesday

BREAKFAST: _____

LUNCH: _____

DINNER: _____

SMOOTHIE OR DESSERT: _____

SNACK: _____

Thursday

BREAKFAST: _____

LUNCH: _____

DINNER: _____

SMOOTHIE OR DESSERT: _____

SNACK: _____

Friday

BREAKFAST: _____

LUNCH: _____

DINNER: _____

SMOOTHIE OR DESSERT: _____

SNACK: _____

Saturday

BREAKFAST: _____

LUNCH: _____

DINNER: _____

SMOOTHIE OR DESSERT: _____

SNACK: _____

Sunday

BREAKFAST: _____

LUNCH: _____

DINNER: _____

SMOOTHIE OR DESSERT: _____

SNACK: _____

Menu Planning Worksheet

Phase 2: Week 6 of Lower Your Blood Pressure Naturally

Monday

BREAKFAST: _____

LUNCH: _____

DINNER: _____

SMOOTHIE OR DESSERT: _____

SNACK: _____

Tuesday

BREAKFAST: _____

LUNCH: _____

DINNER: _____

SMOOTHIE OR DESSERT: _____

SNACK: _____

Wednesday

BREAKFAST: _____

LUNCH: _____

DINNER: _____

SMOOTHIE OR DESSERT: _____

SNACK: _____

Thursday

BREAKFAST: _____

LUNCH: _____

DINNER: _____

SMOOTHIE OR DESSERT: _____

SNACK: _____

Friday

BREAKFAST: _____

LUNCH: _____

DINNER: _____

SMOOTHIE OR DESSERT:_____

SNACK: _____

Saturday

BREAKFAST: _____

LUNCH: _____

DINNER: _____

SMOOTHIE OR DESSERT:_____

SNACK: _____

Sunday

BREAKFAST: _____

LUNCH: _____

DINNER: _____

SMOOTHIE OR DESSERT:_____

SNACK: _____

Shopping List for Phase 2

As in Phase 1, you'll choose your meals in Phase 2. Planning your meals in advance will allow you to figure out which items—and how much—you'll need from the Phase 2 grocery list. Don't forget to check your supply of pantry staples as well. Remember to double, triple, or quadruple amounts as needed if you'd like to prepare extra meals ahead of time or if you're cooking for others.

PHASE 2 SHOPPING LIST

FOOD	WEEK 2	WEEK 3	WEEK 4	WEEK 5	WEEK 6
Condiments					
Cinnamon					
Hummus					
Light mayo					
Reduced-sodium soy sauce					
Salsa (fresh *pico de gallo* style)					
Spice blend recipes (see Chapter 8)					
Fruits					
Apples					
Bananas					
Blueberries					
Kiwifruits					
Peaches/nectarines					
Pears					
Pineapple					
Strawberries					

FOOD	WEEK 2	WEEK 3	WEEK 4	WEEK 5	WEEK 6
Vegetables					
Baby bok choy					
Broccoli					
Cabbage					
Carrots					
Celery					
Cucumbers					
Garlic					
Ginger					
Kale					
Mixed greens					
Mushrooms					
Onion					
Red bell peppers					
Spinach (regular or baby)					
Swiss chard					
Tomatoes					
Fats					
Almond butter					
Almonds					
Avocado					
Sunflower seeds					
Walnuts					

(continued)

FOOD	WEEK 2	WEEK 3	WEEK 4	WEEK 5	WEEK 6
Starches					
Bulgur					
Corn tortillas					
Parsnips					
Potatoes					
Quinoa					
Rolled oats					
Sweet potatoes					
Whole grain and whole wheat bread					
Proteins					
Black beans					
Chicken, boneless, skinless breast or thigh					
Chickpeas					
Eggs					
Halibut					
Kidney beans					
Pork tenderloin					
Shrimp					
Tilapia fillets					
Tofu					
Tuna in olive oil					
White beans					
Dairy					
Fat-free milk or soy milk					

FOOD	WEEK 2	WEEK 3	WEEK 4	WEEK 5	WEEK 6
Feta cheese					
0% plain Greek yogurt					
Fat-free plain (regular) yogurt					
Light vanilla ice cream					
Provolone cheese					
Reduced-fat Cheddar cheese					
Reduced-fat mozzarella cheese					
Swiss cheese					
Other					
Chia seeds					
Cocoa powder					
Coconut flakes					
Dark chocolate					
Gingersnap cookies					
Honey					
Maple syrup					
Orange juice					
Peanut butter					

CHAPTER 10

Dining Out and Convenience Options

Going out to a restaurant with coworkers, family, or your significant other? No time to cook? Grabbing a fast lunch or dinner? On the road for work or vacation, or ferrying a busy family around town? You can feed yourself and your family in a flash without missing out on pressure-lowering minerals or getting an overload of sodium.

When you don't have the time or opportunity to fall back on the recipes in this book, the strategies and meal options in this chapter will help you stay on track. We reviewed the calories, sodium, and mineral levels in hundreds of restaurant entrées, fast-food choices, and healthy packaged foods to find the very best alternatives.

Lightning-Fast Meals at Home

Yes, it can be done! We've coupled healthy, low-sodium convenience foods from the supermarket with mineral-rich fruits, vegetables, and dairy products to create delicious, ready-in-a-flash breakfast, lunch, and dinner options. As you'll see, all provide blood pressure–friendly levels of calcium, magnesium, and potassium while keeping sodium below 500 milligrams and calories close to 350 per serving.

Too Busy to Cook? Stock Up on These

Keep a couple of the frozen (and even canned) main dish entrées recommended in this chapter on hand so you'll always have backup meals for unexpectedly busy nights. Also stock up on the ingredients you'll need to throw together the mineral-rich side dishes that round out each meal. These include:

- Olive oil
- Lemon
- Bananas
- Frozen chopped spinach
- Frozen chopped kale
- Almonds, walnut halves, or sunflower seeds
- Red bell peppers
- Frozen raspberries or peach slices
- A whole grain breakfast cereal with 150 milligrams of sodium or less and 170 calories or less per serving
- Fat-free plain yogurt
- Fat-free milk

If you are going to be busy or don't feel like cooking, keep some of the healthier convenience foods listed ahead on hand, along with the recommended Power Mineral–rich fresh foods. You'll be prepared to eat healthy even when you're on the go, tired, or just feeling lazy.

Quick Breakfasts

Yogurt with Fruit and Nuts: Top 1 cup fat-free plain yogurt with 1 banana, sliced, and 14 walnut halves. Or substitute bananas with 1 cup frozen raspberries or peach slices (thawed) for similar calorie and mineral counts with just slightly less magnesium.

POWER MINERAL TOTALS: 34% calcium, 27% potassium, 27% magnesium

Oatmeal in a Hurry: No time for steel-cut oats? Fall back on old-fashioned oats. In a small saucepan over high heat, bring 1 cup water to a boil and stir in ⅓ cup oats. Return to boil, add 1 cup frozen peaches, cover, and turn off the heat. Go get dressed. In 10 minutes, the oatmeal will be ready. Top with 1 cup fat-free milk and 7 walnut halves.

POWER MINERAL TOTALS: 42% calcium, 22% potassium, 23% magnesium

Cold Cereal and Fruit: Combine 1 serving of your favorite low-sodium breakfast cereal (one with 150 milligrams of sodium or less, such as Kashi GoLean Crisp! or Post Original Shredded Wheat) with 1 cup fat-free milk. Top with ½ banana, sliced, or ½ cup frozen raspberries or peach slices (thawed).

POWER MINERAL TOTALS: 34% calcium, at least 20% potassium, at least 23% magnesium

Fast, Convenient Lunches and Dinners

It's true that most convenience foods are saturated with sodium. But hiding out in this salty landscape are a handful of lower-sodium options that are also low in calories and high in some important minerals. Paired with fresh mineral-rich sides, these fast meals are great for those afternoons and evenings when cooking just isn't going to happen. Each contains about 500 milligrams of sodium or less, possesses around 350 calories, and makes an impressive contribution to your daily intake of Power Minerals. For once-in-awhile eating, these are terrific choices.

Healthy Choice Complete Meals: Herb-Crusted Fish

PAIR WITH: 2 cups raw spinach, diced red bell pepper, 1 teaspoon olive oil, and a spritz of lemon

POWER MINERAL TOTALS: 14% calcium, 27% potassium, 30% magnesium

Healthy Choice Café Steamers: Honey Balsamic Chicken

PAIR WITH: 2 cups raw spinach, diced red bell pepper, 1 teaspoon olive oil, and a spritz of lemon

POWER MINERAL TOTALS: 16% calcium, 35% potassium, 25% magnesium

Healthy Choice Café Steamers: Pineapple Chicken

PAIR WITH: 1 cup kale, steamed, with a spritz of lemon; or microwave 1½ cups frozen chopped kale

POWER MINERAL TOTALS: 22% calcium, 25% potassium, at least 6% magnesium

Healthy Choice Café Steamers: Sweet and Spicy Orange Zest Chicken

PAIR WITH: Small spinach salad: 1 cup raw spinach, diced red bell pepper, ½ ounce nuts or seeds (11 almonds or 7 walnut halves or 1 tablespoon sunflower seeds), 1 teaspoon olive oil, and a spritz of lemon; or microwave ½ cup frozen chopped spinach and top with the other ingredients.

POWER MINERAL TOTALS: 32.5% calcium, 27% potassium, 25.5% magnesium

Amy's Light in Sodium Shepherd's Pie

PAIR WITH: 3 cups raw spinach, ¼ cup diced red bell pepper, 1 teaspoon olive oil, and a spritz of lemon; or microwave 1 cup frozen chopped spinach and top with the other ingredients

POWER MINERAL TOTALS: 19% calcium, 17% potassium, 16% magnesium

Amy's Light in Sodium Brown Rice & Vegetables Bowl

PAIR WITH: 3 cups raw spinach, ¼ cup diced red bell pepper, 1 teaspoon olive oil, and a spritz of lemon; or microwave 1 cup frozen chopped spinach and top with the other ingredients

POWER MINERAL TOTALS: 17% calcium, 17% potassium, 16% magnesium

Amy's Light in Sodium Vegetable Lasagna

PAIR WITH: 3 cups raw spinach, ¼ cup diced red bell pepper, 1 teaspoon olive oil, and a spritz of lemon; or microwave 1 cup frozen chopped spinach and top with the other ingredients

POWER MINERAL TOTALS: 34% calcium, 17% potassium, 16% magnesium

Lean Cuisine Baja-Style Queso Dip with Pita Bread

PAIR WITH: 3 cups raw spinach, ¼ cup diced red bell pepper, ½ ounce nuts or seeds (11 almonds or 7 walnut halves or 1 tablespoon sunflower seeds), 1 teaspoon olive oil, and a spritz of lemon; or microwave 1 cup frozen chopped spinach and top with the other ingredients

POWER MINERAL TOTALS: At least 11% calcium, 19% potassium, 21% magnesium

Lean Cuisine Thai-Style Chicken Spring Rolls

PAIR WITH: 3 cups raw spinach, ¼ cup diced red bell pepper, ½ ounce nuts or seeds (11 almonds or 7 walnut halves or 1 tablespoon sunflower seeds), 1 teaspoon olive oil, and a spritz of lemon; or microwave 1 cup frozen chopped spinach and top with the other ingredients

POWER MINERAL TOTALS: At least 11% calcium, 32% potassium, 21% magnesium

Lean Cuisine Wood Fire Style BBQ Recipe Chicken Pizza

PAIR WITH: 1 cup kale, steamed, with a spritz of lemon; or microwave 1½ cups frozen chopped kale

POWER MINERAL TOTALS: At least 18% calcium, 25% potassium, at least 6% magnesium

Lean Cuisine Honestly Good Lemongrass Salmon or Plum Ginger Grain-Crusted Fish

PAIR WITH: 1 cup kale, steamed, with a spritz of lemon; or microwave 1½ cups frozen chopped kale

POWER MINERAL TOTALS: At least 18% calcium, 25% potassium, at least 6% magnesium

Amy's Organic Light in Sodium Lentil Soup (½ can)

PAIR WITH: 1 cup (8 ounces) fat-free milk plus 2 cups raw spinach, diced red bell pepper, 1 teaspoon olive oil, and a spritz of lemon; or have the milk with 1 cup frozen chopped spinach, microwaved, topped with the other ingredients

POWER MINERAL TOTALS: 39% calcium, 22% potassium, 19% magnesium

Amy's Organic Light in Sodium Medium Chili (½ can)

PAIR WITH: 3 cups raw spinach, ¼ cup diced red bell pepper, 1 teaspoon olive oil, and a spritz of lemon; or microwave 1 cup frozen chopped spinach and top with the other ingredients

POWER MINERAL TOTALS: 29% calcium, at least 17% potassium, at least 16% magnesium

Amy's Organic Light in Sodium Chunky Tomato Bisque (½ can)

PAIR WITH: 3 cups raw spinach, ¼ cup diced red bell pepper, ½ ounce nuts or seeds (11 almonds or 7 walnut halves or 1 tablespoon sunflower seeds), 1 teaspoon olive oil, and a spritz of lemon; or microwave 1 cup frozen chopped spinach and top with the other ingredients

POWER MINERAL TOTALS: 24% calcium, at least 23% potassium, at least 35% magnesium

Campbell's Low Sodium Cream of Mushroom Soup (1 can)

PAIR WITH: 3 cups raw spinach, ¼ cup diced red bell pepper, ½ ounce nuts or seeds (11 almonds or 7 walnut halves or 1 tablespoon sunflower seeds), 1 teaspoon olive oil, and a spritz of lemon; or microwave 1 cup frozen chopped spinach and top with the other ingredients

POWER MINERAL TOTALS: 20% calcium, at least 23% potassium, at least 35% magnesium

Dining Out

In the 21st century, few of us eat at home all the time. On the Lower Your Blood Pressure Naturally plan, you can eat out without overdoing calories or sodium and without skimping on pressure-regulating minerals. Our test panelists did it. They lost weight and lowered their blood pressures while enjoying the occasional lunch out with coworkers or a weekend dinner out with a significant other, family, or friends. Follow our guidelines for discovering low-sodium, low-calorie, mineral-rich menu items and for sidestepping salt-and-calorie bombs. You'll also find specific suggestions for dozens of major American fast-food and casual dining chains in this section.

Eight Rules for BP-Friendly Dining

1. Double up.
On this plan, you'll eat five times a day in Phase 2: four meals plus a smoothie or dessert. If you're having lunch or dinner in a restaurant, consider that meal equal to two of your daily plan meals. This will give you the flexibility to enjoy more calories and a bit more sodium—and more menu options—without straying from the plan. Try to have a smoothie on the day you eat out to help keep your intake of all three Power Minerals as high as possible.

2. Sip simply.
Stick with water, plain unsweetened iced tea, hot tea, or coffee—all of which have zero calories and virtually no sodium. Some sweet drinks, such as certain brands of lemonade, contain up to 100 milligrams of sodium along with empty calories. Think twice about alcohol. According to a 2012 study from Sweden's Uppsala University, it triggers even more overeating than TV watching or trying to get through a long day without enough sleep.[1] Fat-free or 1% milk is a good option if your meal is low in calories and if you haven't already had two servings of dairy for the day.

3. Subtract the salt and multiply the minerals in your salad.
Fresh greens, ripe tomatoes, cucumbers, carrots—a salad is a great, mineral-rich choice as a meal starter or main dish when you're eating out. But high-sodium add-ons can change the picture. These are examples from real restaurant menus: An ounce of crumbled blue cheese can add 381 milligrams of sodium, a shake of bacon bits up to 442 milligrams, and croutons 215 milligrams. Dodge these salt bombs by ordering your salad without them or by removing them when it arrives. Ask for oil and vinegar or a lemon wedge instead of prepared salad dressings, which can contribute an additional 200 to 700 milligrams of pressure-raising sodium!

 If it's an option, order extra vegetables in your salad (as you can at Cosi restaurants). A few slices of avocado or red bell pepper bump up the potassium and magnesium in your meal. A handful of chopped carrot bestows extra potassium. Plain nuts—without salt or sugary coatings—are also a good choice because they bump up the magnesium level of your meal.

Your best bet? A trip to the salad bar, where you can choose fresh raw vegetables for yourself and sidestep salty additions.

4. Enjoy delicious, pressure-friendly gems.

Hiding on many menus are treats that won't blow your sodium or calorie "budget" and that will increase your intake of Power Minerals. Look for plain baked potatoes, which can deliver a big dose of potassium. (If the potato is big, split it with your dining partner; a large spud can deliver 200 calories.) Dress it up with a splash of vinegar or a sprinkle of olive oil. Also keep an eye out for fresh fruit alone or paired with yogurt. Both ways, it's a consistently low-sodium option that's good for your blood pressure. At breakfast, oatmeal's a terrific choice. Add fruit and nuts for flavor and a nutritional boost. Steamed or roasted plain vegetables are usually a good choice, though we were surprised at the high sodium levels in some of these (presumably because the veggies were bathed in a salty solution during cooking). Refer to the restaurant guide starting on page 156 for best options.

5. Zero in on grilled, broiled, or blackened fish.

Simply prepared salmon, tilapia (a Power Food), halibut, and wahoo were consistent top choices for sodium-conscious eaters in our review of restaurant nutrition info. Steer clear of salty toppings, like barbecue glazes, soy or teriyaki sauces, and salsas. Surprisingly, unadorned fish was lower in sodium than grilled skinless chicken on many menus. In our restaurant guide, we often suggest splitting grilled chicken and a salad with a friend to keep the sodium in your meal below 500 milligrams.

6. Know which entrées to skip.

In our review, entrées that tilted our "salt meter" with more than 1,000—often more than 2,000, 3,000, and 4,000!—milligrams of sodium per serving had several things in common. Toppings such as sauces, cheese, mayonnaise, and even salsa equaled more sodium. Fried foods often had higher sodium levels. While some plain meats were lower in sodium, their fat contents made them unwise choices for anyone concerned about heart health. We also found extremely high levels of sodium in almost all soups, almost all appetizers, and in many restaurant and fast-food sandwiches, wraps, and burritos.

7. Banish the bread basket.

Say no to the rolls and biscuits that appear on most restaurant tables soon after you order. These can add hundreds of grams of sodium and plenty of calories to your meal. Turn down the cheesy biscuits, Texas toast, and buttered garlic bread that sometimes accompany entrées and salads. In our check of restaurant nutrition facts, these added 270 to 990 extra milligrams of sodium. Hungry when you sit down? Ask for a plain side salad and dress it with a splash of oil and vinegar.

8. Don't assume that "healthy" equals low sodium.

We found high sodium levels in many vegetarian, vegan, gluten free, and even "fit" or "healthy" options. The exception: Entrées that have earned the American Heart Association's Heart-Check mark: a red heart with a white check mark through it. These contain 700 calories or less and 800 milligrams of sodium or less, are low in saturated fat and cholesterol, and provide 10 percent or more of the Daily Value of one of the following nutrients: vitamin A, vitamin C, calcium, iron, dietary fiber, or protein.

Restaurant Guide

We bet you'd be as shocked as we were when we reviewed nutrition information for dozens of casual dining spots across America. We found beverages with nearly 200 milligrams of sodium, burgers and chicken dishes with more than 3,000 milligrams (way more than the 2,300 milligrams we should get in a day), and soups and salads with a day's worth of sodium. There's even a noodle dish with 6,190 milligrams of sodium, nearly three times the healthy level! Wow!

Hidden among these salt disasters, we found main dishes and sides that keep sodium and calories to a reasonable level and that contain the Power Minerals you need for optimal blood pressure. Remember that if you're going out for lunch or dinner, it's okay to use the calorie and sodium "allowances" that would normally cover two meals on this plan. Eat one less meal from the plan that day. This gives you a budget of about 700 calories and up to 800 milligrams of sodium (the upper limit recommended by the American Heart Association for a single meal). Stick carefully to your plan the rest of the day, of course, so that you can enjoy your meal away from home.

Peruse these recommendations.

Applebee's

Main dishes: Grilled Chicken Caesar Salad, no dressing, ½ portion (180 calories, 450 mg sodium); Caesar Salad, lunch portion, no dressing (210 calories, 350 mg sodium)

Side: Fresh Fruit (90 calories, 0 mg sodium)

Baja Fresh

Tacos: Original Baja Taco with chicken (210 calories, 230 mg sodium) or shrimp (200 calories, 280 mg sodium); Grilled Wahoo Taco (230 calories, 300 mg sodium)

Sides: Guacamole, 3-ounce size (110 calories, 270 mg sodium); Veggie Mix (110 calories, 330 mg sodium)

Bob Evans

Breakfast options: 2 Scrambled Egg Lites (57 calories, 238 mg sodium); 3 Scrambled Egg Whites (75 calories, 269 mg sodium); Fruit and Yogurt Plate (348 calories, 73 mg sodium)

Sides: English Muffin (146 calories, 243 mg sodium); slice of whole wheat toast with margarine (97 calories, 187 mg sodium); Fresh Fruit Dish (58 calories, 7 mg sodium)

Main dishes: Garlic Butter Salmon (256 calories, 174 mg sodium); Salmon (243 calories, 101 mg sodium); Wildfire Salmon (312 calories, 203 mg sodium)

Sides: Steamed Broccoli Florets (34 calories, 33 mg sodium); Fresh Fruit Plate with Low-Fat Strawberry Yogurt (353 calories, 73 mg sodium); Baked Potato with margarine (231 calories, 32 mg sodium); Baked Potato, plain (193 calories, 0 mg sodium); Fresh Fruit Dish (58 calories, 7 mg sodium); Farmhouse Garden Salad, no dressing (76 calories, 126 mg sodium)

Boston Market

Main dishes: Turkey Breast, regular size (180 calories, 620 mg sodium); Corn (120 calories, 55 mg sodium)

Carrabba's

Main dishes: Veal Marsala, small (321 calories, 429 mg sodium); Grilled Salmon, small (478 calories, 521 mg sodium)

Sides: House Salad (278 calories, 374 mg sodium); Sautéed Spinach, plain (26 calories, 354 mg sodium); Cucumber Tomato Salad (115 calories, 118 mg sodium)

Chipotle

Main dishes: Burrito Bowl with black beans, brown rice, fajita vegetables, and lettuce (305 calories, 570 mg sodium); Salad with romaine lettuce, pinto beans, fajita vegetables, and sour cream (265 calories, 505 mg sodium); soft corn tortillas with chicken and fajita vegetables (420 calories, 585 mg sodium); crispy corn tortillas with chicken and fajita vegetables (390 calories, 570 mg sodium)

Cosi

Breakfast options: Oatmeal (149 calories, 47 mg sodium); Fresh Fruit Yogurt Parfait–Strawberry (345 calories, 229 mg sodium); Fresh Fruit Yogurt Parfait– Bananas Foster (419 calories, 238 mg sodium); Mango Mandarin Greek Yogurt Parfait (283 calories, 181 mg sodium)

Add: Fruit Salad (83 calories, 17 mg sodium)

Main dishes: Signature Salad (644 calories, 678 mg sodium); Signature Salad Light (406 calories, 483 mg sodium); Hummus and Veggie Sandwich (417 calories, 552 mg sodium)

Note: Add fresh avocado, grapes, cucumbers, carrots, or pears to salads. Choose baby carrots instead of bread with entrées.

Snacks: Hummus Shareable, ½ portion (339 calories, 416 mg sodium); Brie and Fruit (498 calories, 353 mg sodium)

International House of Pancakes

Breakfast options: Banana and Brown Sugar Oatmeal (260 calories, 35 mg sodium); Create Your Own Omelette with egg substitute (140 calories, 320 mg sodium), add peppers, onions, mushrooms, or tomatoes (10 calories each, 0 mg sodium); Seasonal Mixed Fruit (60 calories, 0 mg sodium)

Olive Garden

Main dish: Herb Grilled Salmon (480 calories, 360 mg sodium)

Sides: Garden Fresh Salad, no dressing (60 calories, 270 mg sodium—adding dressing takes the sodium to 760 mg); Steamed Broccoli from kids' menu (15 calories, 10 mg sodium)

Outback Steakhouse

Main dishes: Perfectly Grilled Salmon (387 calories, 295 mg sodium); Victoria's Filet, 6 ounces (218 calories, 206 mg sodium)

Sides: House Salad (117 calories, 146 g sodium); Sweet Potato (318 calories, 172 mg sodium); Fresh Seasonal Mixed Vegetables (96 calories, 153 mg sodium)

Panera

Breakfast option: Power Breakfast Egg Bowl with Steak (270 calories, 440 mg sodium)

Main dishes: Roasted Turkey & Avocado BLT on Sourdough (250 calories, 490 mg sodium); Asian Sesame Chicken Salad, whole portion (420 calories, 500 mg sodium); BBQ Chicken Salad, whole portion (480 calories, 550 mg sodium); Caesar Salad, whole portion (310 calories, 480 mg sodium); Chicken Caesar Salad, whole portion (440 calories, 660 mg sodium);

Fuji Apple with Chicken Salad, whole portion (550 calories, 620 mg sodium); Spinach Power Salad, whole portion (450 calories, 700 mg sodium); Power Mediterranean Chicken Bowl (360 calories, 430 mg sodium)

Side: Apple (80 calories, 0 mg sodium)

Perkins

Breakfast options: 3-egg omelette with broccoli and mushrooms (245 calories, 335 mg sodium); 3-egg omelette with spinach and tomatoes (220 calories, 245 mg sodium); 3-egg omelette with garden mix (215 calories, 215 mg sodium); 2-egg omelettes also available

Add: Fruit Cup (50 calories, 10 mg sodium); Whole Wheat Toast, no butter (2 pieces in order, 220 calories, 440 mg sodium)

Main dishes: Chef Deluxe Salad, without deli ham, bacon, cheese, and black olives (260 calories, 500 mg sodium); Tilapia Grille, without roll, herb rice, tartar sauce, and butter blend (310 calories, 130 mg sodium); Grilled Salmon, without roll, herb rice, and butter blend (490 calories, 160 mg sodium)

Side: Side Salad (order without croutons, cheese, or dressing to bring count to 20 calories, 15 mg sodium)

P.F. Chang's

Appetizer: 2 Spring Rolls (156 calories, 271 mg sodium)

Main dishes: Eat just half of an order of these (take the rest home or split the meal with a friend): Philip's Better Lemon Chicken (900 calories, 260 mg sodium); Norwegian Salmon Steamed with Ginger (830 calories, 810 mg sodium); Sweet and Sour Chicken Lunch (690 calories, 450 mg sodium); Dali Chicken Lunch (630 calories, 680 mg sodium); Buddha's Feast Steamed Lunch with white rice (440 calories, 160 mg sodium)

Sides: Garlic Snap Peas, large (200 calories, 270 mg sodium); Asian Tomato Cucumber Salad, small (60 calories, 170 mg sodium); brown rice, 6 ounces (310 calories, 5 mg sodium)

Ponderosa

Main dishes: Tilapia (167 calories, 361 mg sodium); Salmon (405 calories, 498 mg sodium)

Sides: Baked Potato, plain (275 calories, 85 mg sodium); Garden Salad, no dressing (60 calories, 88 mg sodium)

Red Lobster

Main dishes: Bar Harbor Salad with shrimp (260 calories, 350 mg sodium) or salmon (350 calories, 135 mg sodium); Grilled Fresh Salmon (250 calories, 480 mg sodium); Blackened Walleye, dinner portion (300 calories, 410 mg sodium); Broiled Walleye, lunch portion (130 calories, 270 mg sodium); Blackened Catfish, lunch portion (190 calories, 150 mg sodium)

Sides: Asparagus (60 calories, 270 mg sodium); Garden Salad (100 calories, 160 mg sodium); Roasted Vegetable Medley (40 calories, 170 mg sodium)

Ruby Tuesday

Main dishes: Plain Grilled Chicken (215 calories, 248 mg sodium); Hickory Bourbon Chicken (275 calories, 438 mg sodium)

Sides: Steamed Broccoli (52 calories, 113 mg sodium); Roasted Spaghetti Squash (54 calories, 69 mg sodium); Baked Potato, plain (259 calories, 103 mg sodium)

Steak 'n Shake

Breakfast options: 2 eggs, scrambled (160 calories, 140 mg sodium); Yogurt Parfait (210 calories, 95 mg sodium)

Main dish: Apple Pecan Grilled Chicken Salad (330 calories, 640 mg sodium)

Uno Chicago Grill

Main dishes: Citrus BBQ Salmon (590 calories, 170 mg sodium); Garden Salad with Grilled Chicken (310 calories, 870 mg sodium—skipping the dressing and croutons will lower the sodium content)

Sides: Brown rice (180 calories, 100 mg sodium); Roasted Seasonal Vegetables (80 calories, 160 mg sodium); Steamed Broccoli (70 calories, 360 mg sodium); Farro Salad (180 calories, 160 mg sodium)

Fast-Food Guide

If you have to grab a meal at a drive-thru or are hankering for a burger once in a blue moon, your best sodium-controlled bet is usually a chain's smallest, plainest burger. Pair it with a side salad—no dressing (ask for a lemon wedge), croutons, or cheese—and a container of milk. The combination will keep your sodium intake at a reasonable level while providing calcium as well as some potassium and magnesium from the salad greens and enriched burger bun. Another easy-to-find option: fruit and yogurt parfaits. These are surprisingly low in sodium and deliver pressure-soothing calcium plus a small dose of magnesium and potassium.

Here are some options to consider when fast food is on your radar.

Arby's

Main dish: Jr. Roast Beef (210 calories, 530 mg sodium)

Side: Chopped Side Salad (70 calories, 105 mg sodium)

Chick-fil-A

Breakfast option: Yogurt Parfait with granola (350 calories, 140 mg sodium)

Main dish: Grilled Market Salad (180 calories, 680 mg sodium)

Sides: Fruit Cup, large (90 calories, 0 sodium); Side Salad (80 calories, 110 mg sodium)

McDonald's

Breakfast options: Fruit & Maple Oatmeal, without brown sugar (260 calories, 115 mg sodium); Fruit 'n Yogurt Parfait (150 calories, 70 mg sodium)

Main dish: Regular hamburger (250 calories, 480 mg sodium)

Drink: 1% Milk (100 calories, 125 mg sodium)

Sonic

Main dish: Jr. Burger (330 calories, 480 mg sodium)

Drink: 1% Milk (110 calories, 130 mg sodium)

Taco Bell

Main dishes: Chalupa Supreme Steak (350 calories, 500 mg sodium); Fresco Crunchy Taco (150 calories, 310 mg sodium); Fresco Grilled Steak Soft Taco (150 calories, 410 mg sodium); Fresco Crunchy Taco (150 calories, 310 mg sodium)

Sides: Black Beans (80 calories, 200 mg sodium); Guacamole (35 calories, 105 mg sodium); Reduced-Fat Sour Cream (30 calories, 20 mg sodium); Salsa Verde (5 calories, 55 mg sodium)

Wendy's

Breakfast options: Steel-Cut Oatmeal with cranberries and pecans, or with summer berries, or with apples and caramel, or plain—all are about 160 calories (except cranberries and pecans, 330 calories) and have 190 to 250 mg sodium

Main dishes: Spicy Chicken Caesar Salad, ½ portion (250 calories, 520 mg sodium); Baked Potato, plain (270 calories, 25 mg sodium), add shredded Cheddar cheese (70 calories, 110 mg sodium)

Side: Garden Side Salad (20 calories, 30 mg sodium)

Drink: 1% Milk (100 calories, 125 mg sodium)

Part III

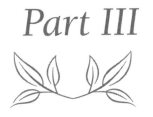

Exercise

At a Glance:
The Workout Plan

This workout plan, based on the latest well-designed research studies, brings together the blood pressure–lowering power of walking, interval training, strength training, yoga, and meditation. We've combined them in a plan that's flexible, easy, and time-saving. Here's what you'll do:

Twenty minutes of higher-intensity interval walking three times per week. For these walks, you'll alternate short bouts of higher-speed walking with your regular pace. Interval walking burns more calories and more body fat, and it has plenty of other health benefits. Best of all, it's a completely customized routine that works no matter what your normal walking pace or fitness level may be. Just going a little faster for short bursts creates the benefits. You can walk outdoors or indoors on a treadmill, or you can substitute another cardio exercise—biking, elliptical training, swimming, even running—if you prefer.

Thirty minutes of moderate walking three times per week. It's okay to break this up into two or even three shorter walks. In fact, studies show that taking a couple of short walks daily keeps blood pressure lower for more hours each day. As with interval walking, you can stroll outdoors, use a treadmill, or substitute another cardio exercise.

A short "blood pressure bonus" routine six times per week. You'll strength train twice a week and do an energizing or restorative yoga work-out 4 days a week. (Just don't strength-train on consecutive days.) In addition, you'll do a 5-minute relaxing meditation daily, fitting it into your day whenever and wherever you want.

One rest day per week. *Ahhhh!* Take a day off every week. You can either schedule a day off or use this free day to stay on track. In other words, if life throws a curveball, and you just don't have a free moment for movement, consider this your rest day and pick up your routine tomorrow.

YOUR 7-DAY PLAN

Use this chart as a guide for planning your workouts. Feel free to swap days according to your schedule, but don't do interval walks or strength-training routines 2 days in a row.

	DAY 1	DAY 2	DAY 3	DAY 4	DAY 5	DAY 6	DAY 7
Interval Walks (20 minutes)	X		X		X		REST
Brisk Walks (30 minutes)		X		X		X	REST
Blood Pressure Bonus	Yoga: Energizing Routine	Strength Training	Yoga: Restorative Routine	Yoga: Energizing Routine	Yoga: Restorative Routine	Strength Training	REST
5-Minute Meditation	X	X	X	X	X	X	X

CHAPTER 11

Workout Plan FAQs

Before you lace up your walking shoes, pick up a hand weight, or flow into your first yoga pose, read this chapter. You'll find all the info you need about exercising safely with high blood pressure as well as advice on proper gear, staying hydrated, working out with weather or time constraints, and more.

Q: Should I get my doctor's okay before exercising?

A: Before you begin any exercise routine, check with your doctor first if you are over age 50, are overweight, don't exercise regularly, have high blood pressure, or have a strong family history of heart disease and don't know your own risk.

If your blood pressure is not under control, it is not safe to start exercising. Talk to your doctor first. If you are under a doctor's supervision for high blood pressure, but it is still not well controlled, do not lift weights, interval train, or perform any yoga moves that include inversions (when your head is lower than your heart) without your doctor's approval. While all of these forms of exercise—walking, strength training, and yoga—are proven to help high blood pressure, they can also temporarily raise your blood pressure. So it's important to take some common-sense precautions. All of the exercises can be modified to work for you, but only with your doctor's okay. Show your doctor the plan so the two of you can discuss specifics and any limits you should set. For example, your doctor may recommend speeding up just a little during interval walks, using lighter weights for strength training, or avoiding inversions during yoga. Be careful of lifting heavier weights or holding your breath during weight lifting. These can increase your blood pressure and add to the amount of stress on your heart.

Q: I have high blood pressure. Is there anything I should watch for during exercise?

A: Yes. Once you have your doctor's okay to work out, the following steps can keep you safe.

Pay attention to how your body is feeling. Monitor your breathing, energy level, and heartbeat. Pay attention to symptoms like headache, visual changes, or chest pain. These can be signs that your blood pressure is dangerously high. Call your doctor immediately. If you are exercising and start to feel unwell or have chest pain or shortness of breath, check in with your doctor before resuming your exercise program.

Don't exercise if you are sick or have a fever. Wait a few days until after all the symptoms of your illness disappear before resuming your exercise program, unless your doctor has given you other directions.

Stop exercising right away and seek medical care if you have any of these:

- Chest pain or tightness
- Dizziness or faintness
- Pain in an arm or your jaw
- Severe shortness of breath
- An irregular heartbeat
- Excessive fatigue
- Pressure or pain in your chest, neck, arm, jaw, or shoulder or any other symptoms that cause concern

Rest and monitor yourself if you feel any of the following symptoms:

- Shortness of breath
- Increasing fatigue
- Heart palpitations or an irregular heartbeat

If you continue to have problems, seek medical care. If you develop a rapid or irregular heartbeat or have heart palpitations, rest and check your pulse after a few minutes. If your pulse is still irregular or above 100 beats per minute, call your doctor for instructions.

Don't ignore pain. If you have chest pain or pain anywhere else in your body, stop what you're doing. (Forget the old adage, "No pain, no gain!") If you perform an activity while you are in pain, you may be doing more harm than good. Ask your doctor or physical therapist for specific guidelines. Learn to "read" your body and know when you need to stop an activity. If you keep exercising through the pain, you are more likely to get injured and not be able to exercise at all.

Get up slowly during strength training and yoga or after exercising on the floor. Some blood pressure medications can cause orthostatic hypotension, temporary low blood pressure that can make you feel dizzy if you stand up quickly.

Skip caffeine. A preworkout cup of coffee may cause a spike in blood pressure. Avoid caffeine 3 to 4 hours before exercising.

Q: Can I adapt the walking program for my favorite form of exercise—jogging, biking, swimming, or using an exercise machine?

A: Absolutely. You can do interval training and steady-paced workouts with any aerobic activity that you enjoy. Just follow the directions for warmups, cooldowns, and what to do in-between. If you use a treadmill, exercise bike, elliptical trainer, stairclimber, or other exercise machine, you can set the resistance to a slightly higher level for the higher-intensity portion of interval workouts or just move faster. If you're swimming, you may want to do a longer warmup to be sure all of your muscles are ready for action and a longer cooldown to ease your heart rate back down.

Q: How can I fit in a workout if it's too hot, too cold, too rainy, or too dark to walk outdoors?

A: Move it to your living room, den, or bedroom. Instead of walking, march in place. For interval workouts, march faster during high-intensity bursts and slower during recovery periods. For steady-paced workouts, just pick a pace that's brisk yet comfortable. You can even watch your favorite TV show while you work out!

Q: I have knee pain. How can I adapt the strength-training and yoga moves to meet my needs?

A: Follow the knee-friendly advice for modifications in these routines. If your knees still hurt, do the strength-training moves standing up or sitting in a chair. Skip any yoga poses that continue to hurt.

Q: I have back problems or occasional back pain. Can I do the strength-training and yoga routines?

A: See your health practitioner if you have concerns about your back. Bring the instructions and photos so she can evaluate which moves and poses are right for you and whether any specific modifications will be needed.

Q: What if I'm really busy and can't fit in a whole walking routine?

A: Do what you can, even if it's sneaking in one or two 5- or 10-minute walks or just getting up and walking around for a few minutes. Any movement is better than no movement! Exercising just for a few minutes can relax and energize you, something you'll appreciate on high-stress days, when you need it most but time is at a premium. And, a growing stack of research shows that just getting up from your desk (or from the couch) every half hour and moving around for 1 to 2 minutes is beneficial. In one 14-year American Cancer Society study, women who sat for 3 or more hours at a time had a 39 percent higher risk of death than those who sat for less time.[1] For every 1 hour of sitting per night, there is an 18 percent increased risk of cardiovascular death and an 11 percent increased risk in overall mortality. Walking to the water fountain, the restroom, around the office, or around your house for a minute or two works the large muscles in your lower body enough to activate a key enzyme that helps pull fats and sugar from your bloodstream.

Q: I like to walk with a friend or two, but they're not interested in interval walks. How can I meet up with my buddies and do the interval routines?

A: Try meeting at a track or walking path that's a loop. Warm up together, split up for the main part of your workout, and then get back together for your cooldown.

Q: Is it better to work out in the morning, the afternoon, or the evening?

A: It all depends on you. Exercising in the morning allows you to get your workout out of the way before the demands of the day can interfere with your plans. But working out later in the day may be more convenient or simply feel better. In one survey, morning exercisers were more likely to stick with their routines than those who scheduled workouts for later on.[2] But other research[3] shows that muscles and joints can be more flexible in the midafternoon—likely because you've already been moving around for several hours, warming up your body. Body temperature is higher then, too. Regardless, the perfect time is the one that works best for you.

Q: What should I look for in walking shoes and socks?

A: The good news is, you don't have to spend a lot to get good walking shoes. In one Scottish study, midpriced shoes were as good as or better than pricey kicks for support, cushioning, and comfort. Look for shoes made for walking, not running. A walking shoe will have a rounded or beveled heel and extra heel cushioning to help support a walker's rolling stride. In contrast, running shoes may have less cushioning in the heel and more in the middle based on the way a runner's foot strikes the ground.

The right socks can also support your workout. Look for types made of wicking material (not cotton) that draw perspiration away from your skin. If you need it, some socks cater to specific needs, providing, for example, extra padding, odor control, or blister-stopping gel cushions.

Get your socks first, and then take them shoe shopping with you. Try on walking shoes late in the day, when feet are bigger (because you've been using them all day!). Have your shoe size and width measured. Test-drive shoes in the store. Walk around or, if you're in a well-appointed walking-shoe store, hop on the treadmill. Walking shoes should feel good right away—no pinching, rubbing, or tight spots.

Q: How should I choose the right weights for the strength-training routine?

A: You don't have to spend a fortune. Look for weights at discount stores (like Walmart, Kmart, or Target) or at shops that sell used exercise equipment. Shop when you have 20 to 30 minutes to try out various weights. And bring along this book.

Know your goal. To find the right hand weights, start by doing one or two of the plan's strength moves with 1- or 2-pound weights. If you can easily do the number of recommended repetitions, move up to slightly heavier weights. If you are new to weight training or if your doctor recommends it, plan on buying lighter weights that you can lift easily. If you're experienced, heavier weights may be better. Choose a set that you can lift with good form for the recommended number of reps.

You can always move up to heavier weights when the moves start to feel easy (and with your doctor's okay, if needed).

Q: How much water should I drink before and during exercise?

A: It's important to stay hydrated. Your body uses water to cool you down, move nutrients around, keep joints lubricated, and maintain healthy blood pressure levels. Have 8 to 12 ounces of water about 10 to 15 minutes before you exercise. Bring a bottle on your walk and sip another 3 to 8 ounces every 15 to 20 minutes, which the American College of Sports Medicine recommends. Have a little more afterward. You don't need a special sports drink; these just add extra calories and are only useful if you're exercising intensely for more than an hour.[4]

CHAPTER 12

The Walking Plan

This is the plan that gives you more for less. Incorporating the proven benefits of high-intensity interval training with the health perks of steady-paced walks, the Lower Your Blood Pressure Naturally walking plan targets your extra pounds, your belly fat, and your blood pressure while saving you time and effort.

You discovered the science behind blood pressure–lowering walking in Part 1. Now it's time to lace up your favorite walking shoes and experience it for yourself. You can also follow this plan while doing other cardio routines—running or swimming or working out on your treadmill, exercise bike, elliptical trainer, stairclimber, or rowing or ski machine.

What You'll Do
1. Take a 20-minute interval walk 3 days a week.
For these walks, you'll alternate short bouts of higher-speed walking with your regular pace. For the first 2 weeks, you'll speed up for 30 seconds and then slow down for a 30-second "recovery period," repeating this interval combo 14 times. The intervals increase to 45 seconds in Weeks 3 and 4 and to 60 seconds in Weeks 5 and 6. It's a completely "customized" routine that works no matter what your normal walking pace or fitness level may be. Just going a little faster for short periods of time activates the benefits. With a warmup and a cooldown included, the whole workout takes just 20 minutes.

2. Take a 30-minute, steady-paced walk 3 days a week.

Walking at a steady, moderate speed for 30 minutes will also help you lose weight, burn fat, and improve your cardiovascular fitness. The time-saving feature: It's okay to break this up into two or even three shorter walks. In fact, studies show that taking a couple of short walks daily keeps blood pressure lower, longer than taking one long walk.

3. Take a break 1 day each week.

That's right; you get a day off. Use it to have some active fun with friends or family, or use it as a fallback in case you missed one of your walks that week. Building in time off helps you stay on track.

What You'll Need

Make sure you have sneakers or walking shoes that fit well and are comfortable. Moisture-wicking socks will keep your feet dry, preventing chafing and blisters. Wear a T-shirt and shorts or workout pants, and add a jacket if it's chilly outside. You'll need a watch or other timepiece to keep track of your time for interval walks. A hat, sunglasses, and a prewalk slathering with sunscreen are smart additions. Carry your cell phone for added safety. If you like listening to music on headphones while you walk, we recommend

---

Walk This Way!

Proper walking form will help you avoid injuries and get the most from your walking routines. Yes, everybody knows how to walk. But the truth is, many people lengthen their strides when they walk faster. This can actually slow you down (your outstretched leg acts like a brake) and puts more stress on your joints and feet, boosting risk for injury.

Instead, take shorter steps. Roll from heel to toes and push off with your toes. Bend your arms (the way runners do). Keep them relaxed and swing them forward and back to a comfortable height (no higher than your chest in front) as you move. This will help you maintain your pace.

---

doing your workouts on a track or walking path—not in places where you'll have to walk in the street or cross streets! Bring a water bottle, especially if you're headed out for a longer walk or it's hot outside. (Turn to Chapter 11 for more advice on walking gear.)

What's Your Intensity Level?

Walking at an intensity that's right *for you* is important. You'll get the most benefits from your own unique pace, which may be slower or faster than you think.

If you're new to exercise or your doctor has suggested that you take it easy, your pace may feel kind of slow. That's okay. Your heart and your waistline will get the most out of your walks when you are consistent. Trying to go too fast increases your risk for injuries. It can also feel bad or stressful, leaving you tempted to stop earlier or to skip more days. Remind yourself that you can always pick up the pace once you have established a regular walking routine and have improved your cardiovascular fitness.

> ## Quick Tip
>
> Tracking your exercise in the logs in Chapter 17 will help you stay motivated.

If you're already exercising regularly (and if your doctor approves), you may have to pick up the pace to get results. Interval walks make your body work harder than usual for short periods of time. You may have to kick it up a notch or two to feel challenged.

Monitoring your intensity level, by using the 1-to-10 perceived exertion scale, will tell you if you're moving at the right pace. It's the easiest way to check in with yourself during exercise because it requires no extra equipment. There's no need for a heart-rate monitor or to stop to take your pulse and do math!

Staying in touch with how your body feels during exercise is an especially important tool for people with high blood pressure. Some blood pressure medications interfere with heart rate, meaning that a heart-rate monitor won't give you an accurate picture of how hard you're working. But the perceived exertion scale (see page 178) will. It's also important to know when to slow down or stop (like if you feel short of breath) and when to get medical help (like if you have chest pain). Tracking your breathing and how you feel during exercise will allow you to do this easily.

The scale goes from 1 (superlow intensity, the way it feels when you're resting on the couch) to 10 (maximum intensity, the way it feels when you are sprinting).

> **Heart Tip**
>
> If you have high blood pressure, review the exercise safety tips in Chapter 11 before you begin the workouts in this plan.

PERCEIVED EXERTION SCALE

EFFORT	INTENSITY	HOW IT FEELS
Resting	1–2	Resting on the couch; waking up in the morning
Easy	3–4	Moving with rhythmic breathing; you can sing
Somewhat hard	5–6	Breathing a bit harder; you can talk in complete sentences
Hard	7–8	Slightly breathless; you can only talk in brief phrases
Very hard	9–10	Breathless. You don't want to talk but you could manage yes/no answers. At a 10, you're working so hard you're gasping for air. No need to get that intense on this plan!

Which Levels Should You Aim for on This Walking Plan?

Ramp up slowly during warmups. Your warmups will take you from Level 1–2 up to a Level 3–4.

During interval walks, pick up the pace in a smart way. If you haven't been exercising regularly or if your doctor recommends that you take it slowly, keep your intensity level lower. Speeding up to an intensity level of 4 and then slowing down to a 3 is fine. (Staying in this range during steady-paced walk days is okay, too.)

We want you to feel good during and after your walks and to look forward to lacing up your walking shoes again tomorrow. As you move through this 6-week plan, increase your intensity level when it feels right for you.

If you are already in good shape and have your doctor's okay (if needed), then challenge yourself. Increase your speed to Level 5 or higher during high-intensity bursts. Experiment to find the intensity level that lets you work hard but also allows you to recharge during recovery periods. You'll know you've picked the right pace if you can hit it during all of the high-intensity bursts.

On interval walks, give yourself a real break during recovery periods. The great thing about interval walks is that you're never far away from the slower pace of recovery periods (when you slow the intensity down). For your recovery pace, aim for a level of 3 to 5. This is the moment where you get to catch your breath before you kick into a higher gear for your next interval. At the end of your recovery period, you should feel rested enough to go fast again. If you're not, dial down the intensity of your fast intervals a little.

Enjoy your breaks; pat yourself on the back for completing the previous interval and get ready to go again. Every time you complete an interval, notice that your confidence is building.

During steady-paced walks, move at your own brisk pace. If you have not been exercising regularly, this could mean a slow stroll—a Level 3 or 4. If you're in great shape, "brisk" might be a Level 7, a pace that only allows you to talk in brief phrases. Choose a level you can sustain for your whole walk. Remember that you can always pick up the pace as your fitness level and strength improve over the course of the 6 weeks.

Cool down slowly and completely. Give your heart, lungs, and muscles time to ease out of exercise mode after your workout. Cool down slowly to a Level 3 or 4. (More on that next.)

Warmups and Cooldowns

Don't be tempted to skip the first 3 minutes or the last 2 minutes of your workout. Starting out slowly warms your muscles and increases the flexibility of joints and connective tissue. It feels good, makes movement easier, and reduces your risk for an injury, all of which add up to a more enjoyable and more effective exercise session.

Warming up raises your body temperature. That alone has a weight loss and fat-burning benefit: For each degree that your body temp rises, your metabolic rate (your body's ability to burn calories) goes up by about 13 percent. As circulation increases, muscles receive more oxygen and fuel. You'll feel energized and notice that switching to a faster pace during your routine seems easier.

Finish your walks by slowing down for the last few minutes. This has several important benefits. During any workout, bloodflow to active muscles increases. Gradually slowing your pace at the end keeps blood from pooling in your legs, which can make you feel a little dizzy or even nauseous.

Cooling down also helps remove a waste product called lactate from your muscles. You'll feel less tired later on. And taking a few minutes to enjoy yourself—and bask in the glow of your exercise "high"—feels great. It's a little bit of "me time" that'll help you look forward to your next walk!

If you have high blood pressure, warmups and cooldowns have additional benefits. Gradually easing into exercise increases your heart rate slowly from a resting state to an active state. It also gives you the opportunity to monitor how you're feeling. You'll have a better sense of what your best pace is today and be less likely to push yourself too hard. Warming up also helps you stay in touch with how you're feeling throughout your walk and catch signs of overexertion early.

Cooling down slowly brings your heart rate and blood pressure back down almost to a resting pace, which is crucial if you have high blood pressure. Don't sit down, stand still, or lie down until you've done your cooldown! If you stop exercising abruptly, your blood pressure can drop too quickly, which can make you feel light-headed or even cause heart palpitations and muscle cramping.

WARMUP AT A GLANCE

Do this 3-minute warmup at the start of every walk (or other cardio activity).

0:00–1:00	Start at an easy pace, whether you are walking outside or using a treadmill, exercise bike, or other cardio machine. If you're walking in place at home, march—lifting your knees and swinging your arms at your sides. If you're jogging or swimming, move at a slow, comfortable speed.
1:01–2:00	Continue walking at a comfortable pace. Reach both arms overhead 20 times. Pump your arms at your sides for the remaining time. You can also do this while jogging, on the treadmill, or, if you have good balance, on an exercise bike. If you're using a machine that also works your arms, like an elliptical trainer or recumbent bike, push and pull the handles more forcefully. If you're swimming, use your arms more vigorously now.
2:01–3:00	Keep moving your legs while pressing your arms in front of you at chest height and then pulling them back so your elbows are pointing behind you, hands by your chest. Do this 20 times. Pump your arms at your sides for the remaining time. Make the same arm movements on a treadmill or exercise bike or while you jog. If you're swimming, switch to backstroke. If you're using a machine with handles, pump your arms a little harder now.

COOLDOWN AT A GLANCE

Do this cooldown at the conclusion of every walk (or other cardio activity). If your heart rate and/or breathing is still fast after 2 minutes, extend your cooldown for another few minutes.

0:00–1:00	Begin slowing your pace gradually. Keep moving your arms. Aim to cut your pace to a Level 4 during the first minute of your cooldown.
1:01–2:00	Slow down to a comfortable stroll. Keep moving your arms. Don't stop or sit down yet. Your breathing and heartbeat should be gradually slowing down. Slow down to a Level 2 or 3, and take more time if needed. Continue moving around for the next 5 to 10 minutes after your walk as you resume your regular activities.

What's Normal, What's Not

Pushing yourself harder feels uncomfortable. Whether you're a beginner starting out with slow walks or an experienced exerciser aiming to bump up the intensity, that uncomfortable feeling means you're challenging yourself to improve your fitness and lose weight. So, some discomfort is normal during exercise. But some signs of discomfort are not normal and mean you should change what you're doing or even stop and get help. Here's what you should know.

HEART RATE

NORMAL: You may feel your heart beating harder and faster.

ABNORMAL: Chest pain, pressure, or tightness; skipped heartbeats, palpitations, or extremely fast heartbeats. What to do: Stop now and call 9-1-1.

BREATHING

NORMAL: You breathe harder and somewhat faster.

ABNORMAL: You're short of breath; breathing is difficult or uncomfortable and doesn't get better when you slow down or stop exercising. What to do: Stop now and call your doctor.

MUSCLES

NORMAL: Some soreness, discomfort, and burning.

ABNORMAL: Sharp, shooting muscle or joint pain. What to do: Stop and rest. Ice the spot when you get home. If the pain continues, call your doctor.

ENERGY LEVEL

NORMAL: Feeling somewhat fatigued during and after your workout.

ABNORMAL: Feeling light-headed, dizzy, or extremely fatigued. What to do: Stop and call your doctor. Call 9-1-1 if symptoms are severe.

Interval Walk Workouts

How often: Three times a week. Alternate with steady-paced walks. Don't do interval walks 2 days in a row. Your muscles need time to recover for best results.

What to do: Warm up. Then begin your intervals. (For about 15 minutes, you'll alternate between faster-paced and slower-paced activity.) After that, cool down. Each walk takes a total of 20 minutes.

What to expect: You'll do longer intervals of high-intensity and low-intensity activity as the weeks go on. If and when you feel ready, you can also increase the intensity.

INTERVAL WALK CHART FOR WEEKS 1 AND 2

ACTIVITY	DURATION	INTENSITY	TIME
Warmup	3 minutes	Gradually increase your intensity from 1 to 3	0:00–3:00
Intervals	Fast pace: 30 seconds	Set by you; could be between 4 and 8	3:01–3:30
	Recovery pace: 30 seconds	3–5	3:31–4:00
	Repeat intervals 14 more times		4:01–18:00
Cooldown	Slow pace: 2 minutes	Gradually decrease your intensity from 3 to 1; take more time to cool down if needed	18:01–20:00

INTERVAL WALK CHART FOR WEEKS 3 AND 4

Increase your faster and slower intervals. Keep moving at the best pace for you. Results come when you're consistent, not by overdoing it. That said, if you're an experienced exerciser, choose a pace that feels challenging. Aim for an intensity level of 6 or higher and see how you feel.

ACTIVITY	DURATION	INTENSITY	TIME
Warmup	3 minutes	Gradually increase your intensity from 1 to 3	0:00–3:00
Intervals	Fast pace: 45 seconds	Set by you; could be between 4 and 8/9	3:01–3:45
	Recovery pace: 45 seconds	3–5	3:46–4:30
	Repeat intervals 9 more times		4:31–18:00
Cooldown	2 minutes	Gradually decrease your intensity from 3 to 1; take more time to cool down if needed	18:01–20:00

INTERVAL WALK CHART FOR WEEKS 5 AND 6

Intervals are a little bit longer now (also, note that the warmup drops to 2 minutes for these walks). Keep monitoring how you feel. Slow your pace enough between brisk intervals so that you feel refreshed when it's time to pick up the pace again.

ACTIVITY	DURATION	INTENSITY	TIME
Warmup	2 minutes	Gradually increase your intensity from 1 to 3	0:00–2:00
Intervals	Fast pace: 60 seconds	Set by you; could be between 4 and 8/9	2:01–3:00
	Recovery pace: 60 seconds	3–5	3:01–4:00
	Repeat intervals 7 more times		4:01–18:00
Cooldown	2 minutes	Gradually decrease your intensity from 3 to 1; take more time to cool down if needed	18:01–20:00

Steady-Paced Walks

How often: You'll take a steady-paced brisk walk three times a week. Alternate with interval walks.

What to do: Warm up, walk at a steady pace, and then cool down. Each walk lasts 30 minutes. It's fine to split up your steady-paced walks into two or three short walks, 10 to 15 minutes each, throughout the day. Research shows that this approach can keep blood pressure lower, longer during the day, and it buffers you from blood pressure spikes, too.

What to expect: Increase your speed as the weeks go on when you feel ready. For your steady-paced walks, aim for an intensity level between 3 and 7. Go slower if you're new to exercise or if your doctor has recommended that you take it easy. Pick up the pace if you are fit and have your doctor's okay (if needed). Invite a friend or family member to join you!

STEADY-PACE WALK CHART FOR WEEKS 1–6

ACTIVITY	DURATION	INTENSITY	TIME
Warmup	3 minutes	Gradually increase your intensity from 1 to 3	0:00–3:00
Brisk-paced walk	25 minutes	3–7	3:01–28:00
Cooldown	2 minutes	Gradually decrease your intensity from 3 to 1; take more time to cool down if needed	28:01–30:00

CHAPTER 13

Daily Blood Pressure Bonus: Build Muscle, Get Energized, Find Serenity

In addition to walking 6 days a week on the Lower Your Blood Pressure Naturally plan, you'll invest 15 minutes a day in a "blood pressure bonus" that promotes healthy numbers in unique and powerful ways. Twice a week, you'll do an easy strength-training routine using hand weights. Four times a week, you'll enjoy either an energizing or restorative yoga routine.

Like our interval walk workouts, these blood pressure bonus routines were developed by *Prevention* magazine fitness editor and registered yoga teacher Jenna Bergen, RYT. Jenna designed all three (there's one strength routine and two different yoga routines) to make the most of your time. You'll be amazed at the difference your 15-minute bonus makes by using strength moves that work multiple muscle groups and yoga positions that effectively energize and relax you. The exercises and poses are easy for beginners to master yet still worthwhile if you're an old hand.

Strength training and yoga contribute to healthier BP in very different ways. But both help reverse invisible, cell-deep conditions that fuel high blood pressure.

Strength training helps you get back muscle mass lost naturally to aging (and to sedentary living). Building sleek, sexy, strong muscle boosts your metabolic rate—your body's ability to burn calories 24/7—making weight loss and weight maintenance much easier. Research suggests that strength training may help keep arteries more flexible, too.

Yoga eases chronic stress, dialing back your body's fight-or-flight response and reducing levels of stress hormones that rev up blood pressure. And by reducing stress, yoga makes it easier for you to make healthier choices throughout the day. (No more grabbing a doughnut or cola when tension's high.) You may find that you sleep better at night, as well, which also helps your BP.

Worth 15 minutes a day? Definitely! Here's what you'll do:

1. **Strength train 2 days a week.** Do this routine on nonconsecutive days, leaving at least 1 day between sessions to allow your muscles to rest, recover, and rebuild. (Do yoga or use your rest day in-between strength-training days.) You'll choose weights that are right for you—lighter or heavier to suit your needs. The six exercises in this routine target several muscles at once, letting you get more done in less time.

2. **Do yoga 4 days a week.** Choose our energizing routine, a great way to get ready for the day, or our restorative routine, a terrific way to wind down in the evening or tame tension any time. Both routines are designed to be safe for people with high blood pressure. We've added modifications to help if you have limitations like joint pain or stiffness.

Blood Pressure Considerations

If you have high blood pressure, talk with your doctor before doing yoga or lifting weights. If you have uncontrolled hypertension (generally a reading of 160/100 or higher), do not exercise without your doctor's approval and guidance. And follow these smart steps to get the most benefits.

- **Read the directions before you try a move or pose.** Using proper form keeps you safe from injuries.

- **Never hold your breath.** Breathe easily and continuously during strength-training moves and yoga poses. Holding your breath during exertion can trigger a spike in your blood pressure.

- **Choose lighter weights.** Heavier weights make your muscles and cardiovascular system work harder, which is great for fitness and muscle building, but will increase your blood pressure more during exercise. If you have high blood pressure, talk with your doctor about the right weights for you. You'll still get results using lighter weights.

- **Skip some yoga poses.** Inversions (such as headstands, shoulder stands, and forward bends) may raise your blood pressure, so it's best to avoid them. You will not find those moves in this plan anyway. The yoga sequences here were mindfully created to avoid poses that are known to increase blood pressure; however, it's best to check with your doctor to make sure you're healthy enough for yoga before starting.

- **Pay attention to how you're feeling.** Stop right away if you become severely out of breath or dizzy or you experience chest pain or pressure. If a yoga pose doesn't feel right for you—if it feels painful or too difficult—try the suggested modifications.

The Strength Workout

You'll use 2- to 12-pound dumbbells for the moves in this routine. For each exercise, use a weight that is heavy enough so that it's challenging to complete the last rep of each set with correct form. However, if you cannot complete your set with correct form, use a lighter weight. If you're new to weight training, choose lighter weights. For advice on choosing the right weights, see Chapter 11.

How often: Twice a week, but not 2 days in a row. Leave a day or two in-between each strength workout. If you'd like to do the routine three times a week, that's fine; just make sure it's on nonconsecutive days.

How long: Do 2 or 3 sets of 10 to 12 repetitions of each exercise unless otherwise noted.

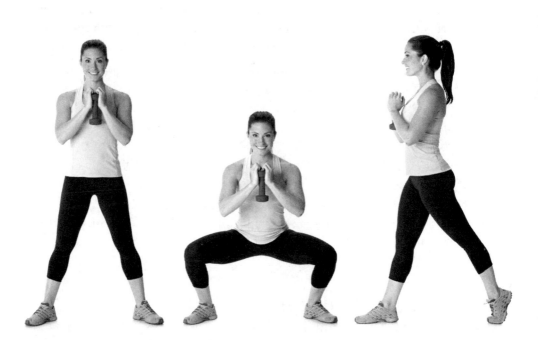

GOBLET SQUAT AND TWIST

Targets: *Butt, thighs, core*

Stand with your feet hip-width apart and hold one dumbbell vertically in both hands in front of your chest, elbows bent and pointing toward the floor. Bend your knees and push your hips back until your thighs are parallel to the ground, lowering into a squat. As you stand, pivot both feet 90 degrees to the right, lifting your left heel. Rotate back to the center and immediately complete another rep, this time rotating to the left. Continue alternating sides with each rep.

MAKE IT EASIER: Omit the twist and/or the weight. If you have back issues, do a simple wall slide instead of a Goblet Squat: Stand with your back against a wall and your feet hip-width apart and about a foot in front of you. Slowly bend your knees, sliding your back down the wall until your thighs are nearly parallel to the ground. (To put less strain on your knees, bend them to about a 45-degree angle.) Pause; then straighten your legs to come back to standing. That's 1 rep.

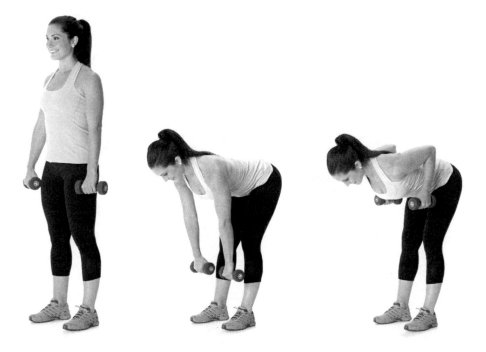

STRAIGHT-LEG DEADLIFT TO ROW

Targets: *Shoulders, back, butt, hamstrings*

Stand with your feet hip-width apart, knees slightly bent, holding one dumbbell in each hand in front of your thighs, palms facing your body. Keeping your back straight, hinge at your hips and lower the dumbbells past your knees, bringing your torso nearly parallel to the floor. Bend your elbows and pull the dumbbells toward your chest. Reverse the move and come back to standing. That's 1 rep.

MAKE IT EASIER: To take pressure off of your lower back, put a deeper bend in your knees and step your feet farther apart.

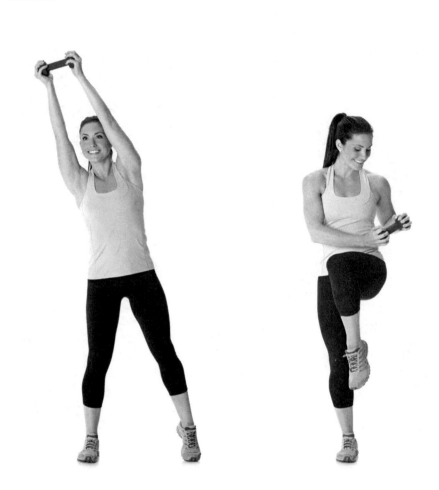

STANDING KNEE LIFT CRUNCH

Targets: *Legs, shoulders, triceps, core*

Stand with your left leg extended a few feet away from your body, left toes on the floor and heel lifted, arms extended over your right shoulder, holding one dumbbell with both hands. Raise your left knee and pull the dumbbell down and across your body. Return to the starting position, quickly moving into the next rep. Finish the reps and repeat on the opposite side to complete 1 set.

MAKE IT EASIER: If you have back issues, don't lower the dumbbell past the point (about chest level) where your torso starts to bend.

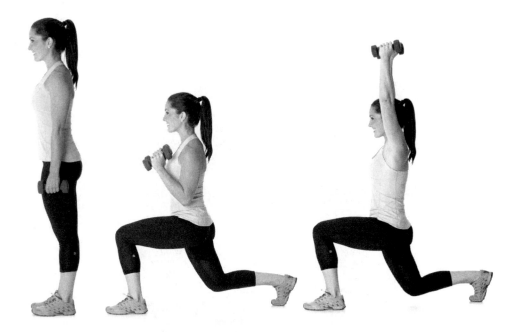

HAMMER CURL LUNGE TO OVERHEAD PRESS

Targets: *Butt, thighs, shoulders, biceps, triceps*

Stand with your feet hip-width apart, holding one dumbbell in each hand at your sides, arms straight and palms facing your body. Step forward with your left foot and lower into a lunge, bending your left knee 90 degrees. As you lunge, curl the dumbbells toward your chest. Holding the lunge, press the dumbbells overhead, extending your arms by your ears. Push yourself back to standing, and then lower the weights to your sides to complete 1 rep. Alternate legs with each rep.

MAKE IT EASIER: Omit the shoulder press. If you have trouble balancing, use a chair. Stand in a split stance, your right leg 2 to 3 feet in front of your left leg, resting your right hand on the back of a chair and holding one dumbbell in your left hand at your side, arm straight and palm facing your body. Lower into a lunge as you curl the dumbbell toward your chest. Holding the lunge, press the dumbbell overhead, extending your arm by your ear. Straighten your legs, then lower the dumbbell to your side to complete 1 rep. Alternate sides for each set.

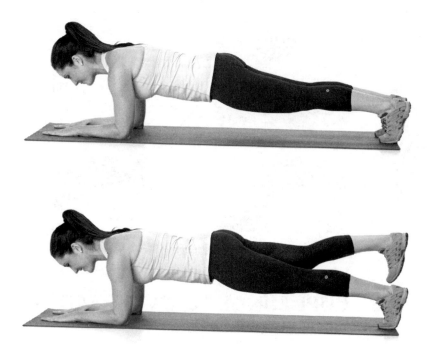

FOREARM PLANK WITH LEG LIFT

Targets: *Butt, core, arms*

Start in a modified pushup position, your weight resting on your forearms and toes, elbows beneath your shoulders, palms flat and shoulder-width apart, abs engaged. Hold for 10 seconds. Lift your right foot a few inches off the floor and hold for 5 seconds. Return your right foot to the floor. Lift your left foot a few inches off the floor and hold for 5 seconds. Return your left foot back to the floor and attempt to hold the plank for 10 more seconds. Release out of the pose and rest for 30 seconds to 1 minute. Repeat one or two more times.

MAKE IT EASIER: Omit the leg lifts. Or do a modified forearm plank: Drop your knees to the floor, making sure to keep your back straight.

HALO SQUAT WITH CHEST PRESS

Targets: *Butt, thighs, shoulders, triceps*

Stand with your feet wider than hip-width apart, toes pointing out, holding one dumbbell with both hands horizontally in front of your chest. Bend your knees and lower into a plié squat, keeping your back straight and your torso over your hips. Circle the dumbbell clockwise around your head. After completing a rotation, press the dumbbell forward, extending your arms at chest height. Reverse the move, pulling the dumbbell back to your chest and then circling it counterclockwise around your head. Continue to change directions with each rep. Try to hold the squat throughout the full set.

MAKE IT EASIER: If your legs get tired, come back to standing and continue with your arms only. Or omit the plié squat altogether and do halos with chest presses while standing. If your arms get tired, omit the chest press and focus on halos only.

Yoga

These two 15-minute routines will relax and energize you. You'll need comfortable, snug-fitting clothing and bare feet. You'll be more comfortable doing the routine on a yoga mat; it keeps you off the floor, provides a little cushioning, and has a grippy surface that helps you hold the poses. You'll also need a yoga block for the energizing routine and a strap or towel for the restorative routine. Have a blanket or pillow nearby if you'd like extra padding, which may be especially useful if you have achy joints. Your favorite music is a nice addition. It can make your practice feel fun and playful.

How often: Do yoga four times a week on the plan. You can do the same routine all four times or mix them up.

What to do: Move slowly through the poses, doing the recommended number of repetitions for each one. During every repetition, hold the pose for a few seconds as you breathe calmly and steadily.

Focus on your breath throughout this routine. Slowly inhale and exhale through your nose, trying to match the length of each inhale to the length of each exhale (about four counts for each). Remember that it may take you a few weeks until you start to feel comfortable and confident in each pose. Flexibility and strength take time to develop. Just focus on your breath, take it slow, and enjoy connecting with your body. Soon the poses will feel like second nature.

Remember to always listen to your body. If a pose hurts, try the modification. If it still hurts, skip that pose and move on to the next one. Yoga is about feeling good and making the poses work for your body.

Energizing Routine

This routine is a wonderful, noncaffeinated way to start each day. It warms and loosens any muscles that may have gotten stiff and achy overnight, and it invigorates your mind and body so you can start the day with focused energy and a positive outlook.

Important note: If you have extremely high/uncontrolled blood pressure, we recommend skipping this routine and doing the restorative one instead. The energizing routine includes several mild inversions that can bring your head lower than your heart. If you would like to try it, get your doctor's approval first.

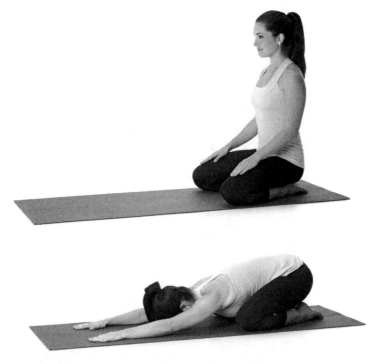

CHILD'S POSE

Start by kneeling on your mat with your big toes touching and your knees spread mat-width apart. Slowly start to walk your hands forward, lowering your torso between your knees and bringing your forehead to rest on the mat. Extend your arms in front of you, allowing your palms to connect with the mat, as you press your tailbone down toward your heels. Bring your attention to your breath, starting to inhale and exhale through your nose. Take a moment to tune in to your body. (Where do you feel tight? Are you feeling relaxed or stressed?) Breathe deeply, holding the pose for 1 minute.

MODIFICATION: If Child's Pose feels uncomfortable, place a folded towel or blanket under your knees for extra cushioning. You can also rest your torso on a pillow, a few folded towels or blankets, or a yoga bolster. In this modification, bring your arms by your sides, palms facing up.

Note: This is a very mild inversion. If you have extremely high blood pressure, you can skip Child's Pose or you can kneel on the floor and sit up, with your back straight and your arms folded in your lap, while breathing deeply for 1 minute.

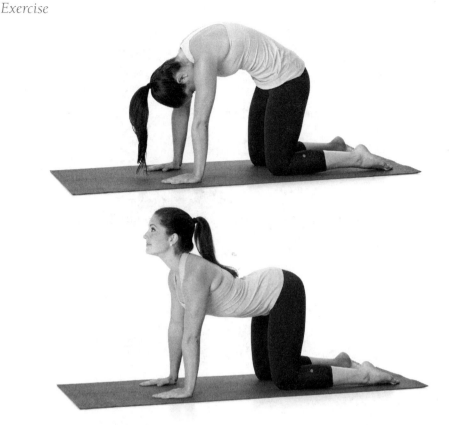

CAT-COW POSE

Slowly come up on all fours, your wrists under your shoulders and your knees under your hips. Inhale, then exhale as you move into the "cat" part of the pose: Round your back toward the ceiling, allowing the crown of your head to release down toward the mat. Inhale as you reverse into the "cow" part of the pose: Lift your chest toward the ceiling and allow your belly to relax and sink toward the floor. Continue to move with the rhythm of your breath, repeating four times and enjoying the delicious stretch in your upper back.

MODIFICATION: If your knees hurt, place a folded towel or blanket under them for extra cushioning.

Note: This is also a very mild inversion. If you have extremely high blood pressure, skip the "cat" part of the pose and just do the "cow" segment—gently lifting your chest toward the ceiling and letting your belly relax. Keep your head lifted and look straight ahead. Breathe in and out eight times.

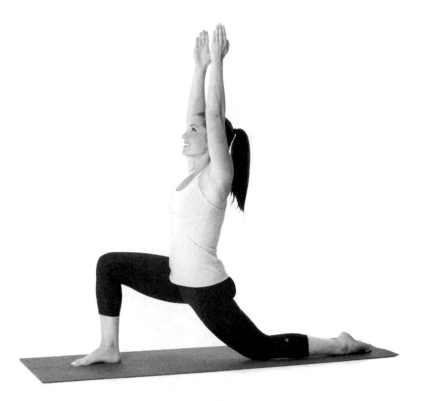

MODIFIED CRESCENT LUNGE TO HAMSTRING STRETCH

From all fours, step your right foot to your right hand and rest the top of your left foot on the mat. Inhale and reach your arms to the ceiling, your biceps by your ears and palms facing inward, as you tuck your tailbone under, feeling a stretch in your left hip flexor. Hold for 30 seconds, breathing deeply. Bring your hands down to the mat on either side of your right foot and slowly press your hips back, keeping your left foot as is but straightening your right leg for a hamstring stretch. Hold for 30 seconds, breathing deeply. Come back to all fours and repeat both stretches on the opposite side.

MODIFICATION: Instead of raising your arms, rest your hands on your right thigh. Place a folded towel or blanket under your left knee.

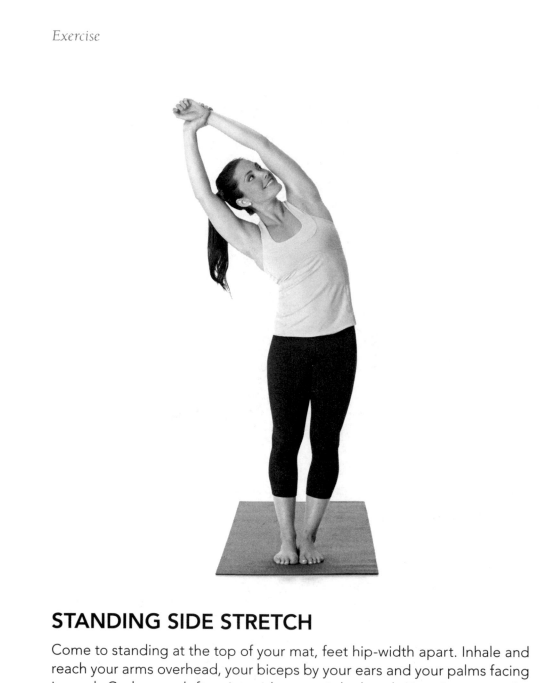

STANDING SIDE STRETCH

Come to standing at the top of your mat, feet hip-width apart. Inhale and reach your arms overhead, your biceps by your ears and your palms facing inward. Grab your left wrist with your right hand. Keeping your abs engaged, exhale and lean your torso to the right, feeling a nice stretch along the left side of your body. Hold here for a few breaths. Come back to standing and repeat the stretch on the opposite side.

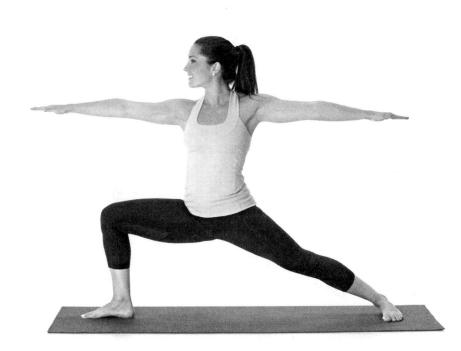

WARRIOR II

From Warrior I, slowly shift your hips, torso, and shoulders to face the left side of the room. Set your left foot parallel to the back of your mat. Bring your right arm toward the front of the room and your left arm toward the back of the room at shoulder height, palms facing down. Keep your shoulders relaxed and centered over your hips. Don't lean your torso forward over your right thigh. Gaze over your right fingertips. Hold for 1 minute, breathing deeply.

MODIFICATION: Don't sink as low in your front knee. If your arms get tired, bring your hands to your hips for a few breaths. You can also take mini breaks by straightening the front leg for a few seconds before coming back into Warrior II.

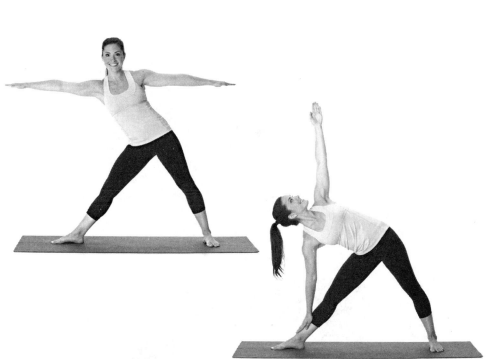

TRIANGLE POSE

From Warrior II, straighten your right leg. Reach through your right finger-tips and lean your torso forward slightly. Hinge at your hips to extend your torso over your right leg, lowering your right hand to rest on your shin or ankle (or on a yoga block outside of your right shin) while extending your left arm upward, aligning your left shoulder over your right shoulder. Keep your head in a neutral position or turn it toward the ceiling to gaze at your left thumb. Hold for 1 minute, breathing deeply. (Partway through your hold, if it feels good, reach your left arm toward the front of the room, your pinky finger spinning down toward the mat, your bicep by your ear, feeling a nice stretch along the side of your body.) Allow your left arm to pull you back to standing. Lower your arms by your sides and step your left foot up to meet your right foot, returning to standing at the front of your mat.

Repeat Warrior I, Warrior II, and Triangle Pose on your opposite side (begin Warrior I by stepping back with your right foot) before completing the rest of this sequence.

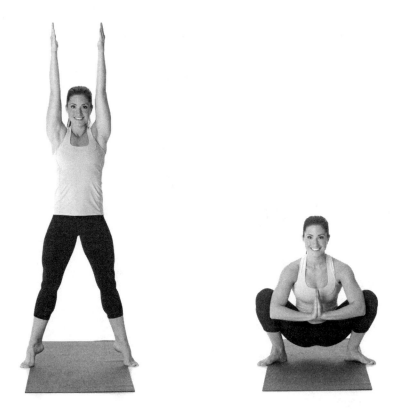

YOGI SQUAT

Stand with your feet wider than hip-width apart, your toes off the mat and your heels on the mat. Inhale and reach your arms overhead, your biceps by your ears and your palms facing inward, lifting your heels and coming up onto the balls of your feet. Exhale and drop your heels to the mat, bend your knees, and lower into a squat, bringing your palms together at heart's center. Press your elbows against your inner knees, feeling a stretch in your inner thighs. Keep your back straight and your belly engaged. Hold for a few seconds. Inhale and straighten your legs, coming back to standing, lifting your heels and balancing on the balls of your feet, as you reach your arms overhead. Exhale and lower back into your squat. Hold here for 30 seconds, breathing deeply.

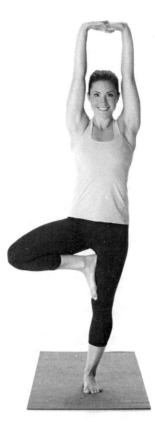

TREE POSE

Inhale and come back to standing with your feet hip-width apart and your arms by your sides. Focus your gaze on a steady point on the floor or the wall in front of you (this will help you balance). Shift your weight onto your left foot and place the sole of your right foot inside your left thigh (never place your foot directly on your knee). When you have your balance, bring your palms together in front of your chest in prayer position. Hold here, or interlace your fingers and press your palms forward, extending your arms at chest height, and then raise your arms overhead. Balance here for 30 seconds to 1 minute, keeping your shoulders relaxed and away from your ears, belly engaged. Repeat Tree Pose on the opposite side.

MODIFICATION: Place the sole of your foot against your inner calf or place your heel on your inner ankle, using your toes as a kickstand.

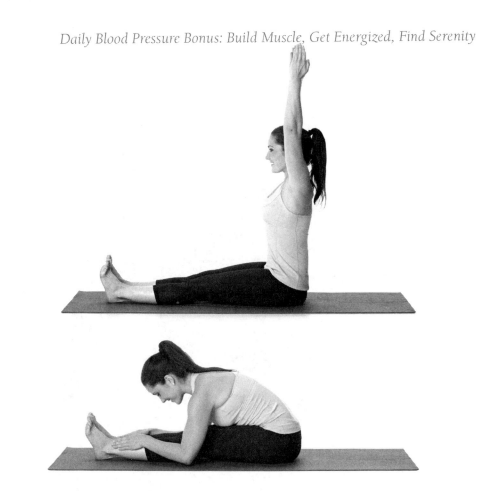

FORWARD FOLD

Sit on your mat with your legs extended in front of you, feet flexed and spine straight. Inhale and raise your arms overhead. Exhale and fold forward, hinging at your hips and bringing your hands to rest on your legs (depending on your flexibility, this may be your thighs, your shins, or even your feet). Don't round your back. Keep lengthening through your spine, reaching the crown of your head toward the wall in front of you. Hold for at least 30 seconds, breathing deeply.

Note: If you have extremely high blood pressure, modify this pose. Sit on the floor as described above. Inhale and reach your arms overhead, and then bend forward, hinging at the hips, until you are about one-third to one-half of the way between sitting straight up and resting your body on your legs. Feel the stretch in your back and in the back of your legs as you breathe out. Hold for as long as you're comfortable, then slowly bring your arms down and your torso back up to sitting straight.

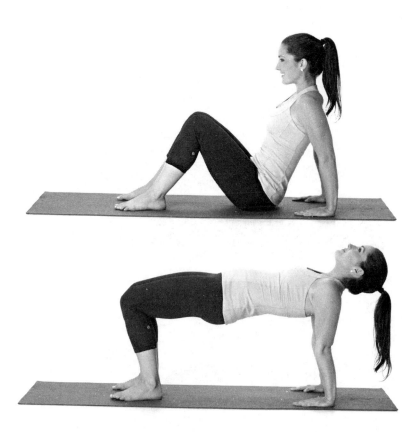

REVERSE TABLE POSE

Bend your knees and bring your feet hip-width apart flat on the mat, hands by your hips with your fingers facing forward. Inhale and press your feet into the mat, lifting your hips toward the ceiling, attempting to get your torso parallel to the floor. (Never force the pose; only lift your hips as high as your body allows.) Allow your head to drop back, feeling a nice stretch in your shoulders. Hold for a few breaths, and then release out of this stretch and slowly lie down on your mat.

MODIFICATION: If you are having trouble lifting your hips, prop them up with a yoga block or a few folded towels or blankets. As you get stronger, you'll be able to do the pose without props.

Note: If you have extremely high blood pressure, skip this pose.

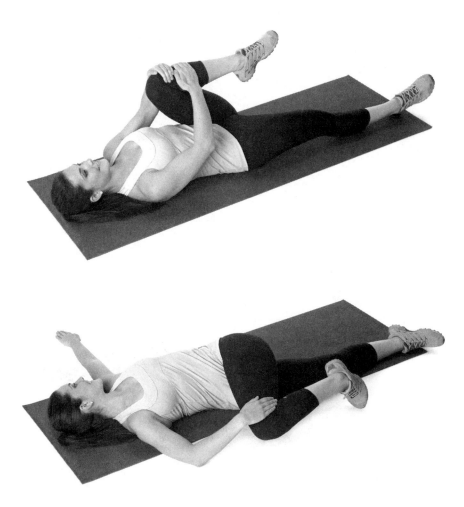

EASY SPINAL TWIST

Lie faceup on your mat with your legs extended and your arms by your sides. Inhale and pull your left knee into your chest. Exhale and bring your left knee across your body toward the right side of the room while keeping your shoulder blades on the floor. Then extend your left arm straight out from your shoulder and gaze over your left fingertips. Hold for 30 seconds, breathing deeply. Repeat on the opposite side.

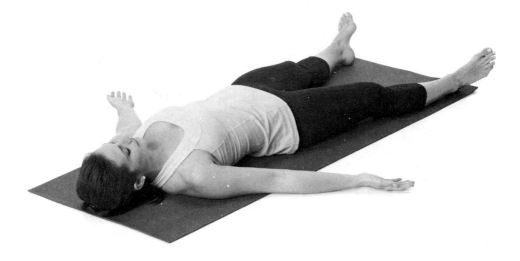

CORPSE POSE

Lie on your back with your legs extended and your arms by your sides, palms facing up. Close your eyes and breathe normally, allowing yourself to relax. Hold for 2 minutes, melting your body into the floor. Roll onto your right side and push yourself up to a seated position to end your practice.

Restorative Routine

Ending your day with a few calming yoga poses is a wonderful, all-natural sleep aid. So find a cozy spot, light a few candles, and enjoy.

What you'll need: A basic yoga mat and a strap or towel; pillows and blankets for extra cushioning are optional.

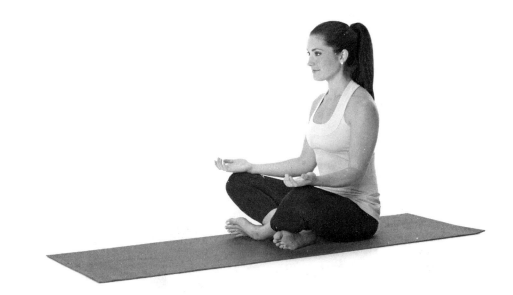

EASY POSE

Come to a seated position with your knees bent and your feet flat on the floor. Wrap your arms around your knees and pull your knees into your chest to help you straighten your spine, sitting up nice and tall. Cross your legs and let your knees fall out to the sides. Rest the backs of your hands lightly on your knees, palms facing up. Close your eyes and start to focus on your breath. Try to clear your mind of all thoughts and worries. Hold here, breathing deeply, for at least 1 minute, eventually working up to 5 minutes, allowing the stress of your day to melt away.

Note: If your hips are tight, you may find that sitting on a folded towel or blanket is more comfortable.

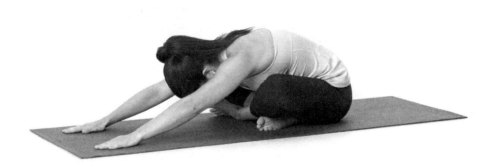

SEATED STRETCH

Keeping your legs crossed and your tailbone connected with the mat, slowly walk your hands forward until your arms are extended in front of you, palms facing down. Bring your forehead to rest on the mat. Hold for at least 1 minute, breathing deeply. Slowly walk your hands back toward you, coming back to a seated position.

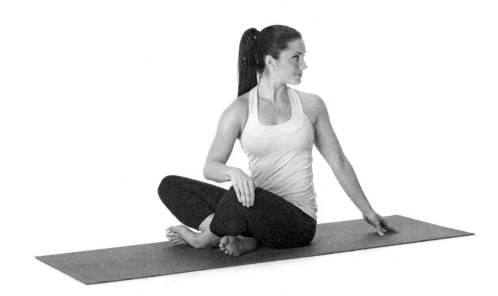

SEATED SPINAL TWIST

Keeping your legs crossed and your tailbone connected with the mat, slowly bring your right hand to the outside of your left knee and place your left palm on the mat beside your left hip. Gently press your right palm into your right knee and twist your torso to the left, bringing your gaze to your left shoulder. Keep your spine long and your shoulders away from your ears. Hold the twist, breathing deeply, for 30 seconds. Release and repeat the twist on the opposite side.

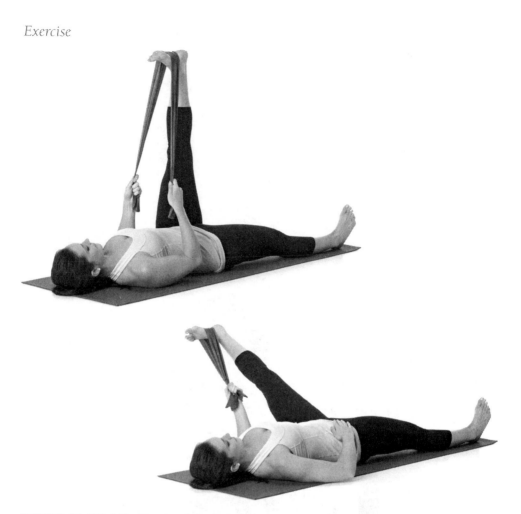

RECLINING BIG TOE POSE

Lie faceup on the mat, legs extended in front of you with feet flexed. Pull your left knee into your chest and hug your thigh to your belly, actively pressing your right leg into the floor. Loop a strap (or a towel) around the arch of your left foot, holding one end of the strap in each hand. Inhale and straighten your left knee, pressing your left heel toward the ceiling, your leg perpendicular to the floor. Hold here, breathing deeply, for 1 minute. If it feels good, take both ends of the strap in your left hand and lower your left leg out to the left and down toward the floor, feeling a stretch in your inner thigh, holding for 30 seconds. Raise your left leg back to the ceiling. Bend your left knee and release out of the stretch. Repeat the pose on the opposite side.

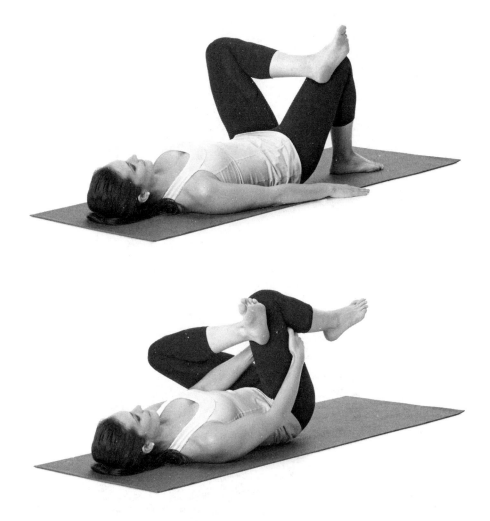

EYE OF THE NEEDLE

Lie on your back with your knees bent and your feet flat on the mat. Cross your left ankle over your right thigh, flexing your left foot. Raise your right knee toward your chest, threading your left arm through the triangle you created with your left leg, and clasp your hands around the back of your right thigh. Try to keep your shoulder blades on the floor as you pull the right knee closer to your chest, simultaneously pressing your left knee away from you. You should feel a deep stretch along the outer left hip. Hold for 1 minute. Release and repeat on the opposite side.

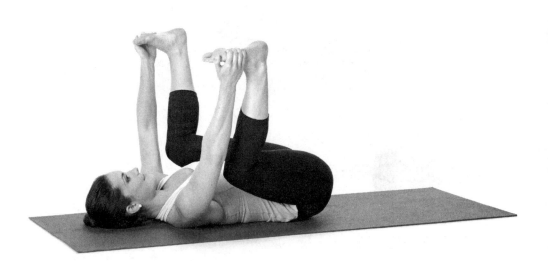

HAPPY BABY POSE

Pull your knees into your chest. Place your hands on the outsides of your feet, opening your knees wider than your torso. Press your feet into your hands while pulling down on your feet, creating resistance. Breathe deeply, holding for 1 minute. If it feels good, rock side to side to massage your lower back.

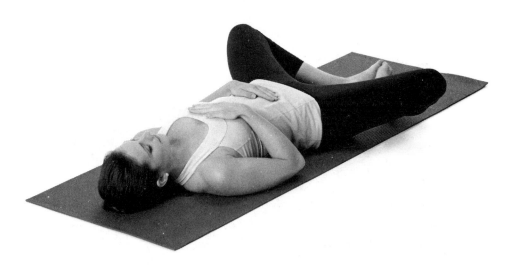

RECLINING BOUND ANGLE POSE

Lie on your back with your legs extended and your arms by your sides, palms facing up. Bend your knees and bring the soles of your feet together, allowing your knees to fall out to the sides. (If it feels good, you can support your knees with folded blankets or towels.) Rest one hand on your chest and the other on your belly. Close your eyes and breathe deeply. Hold for 1 minute to start, gradually increasing to 5 minutes.

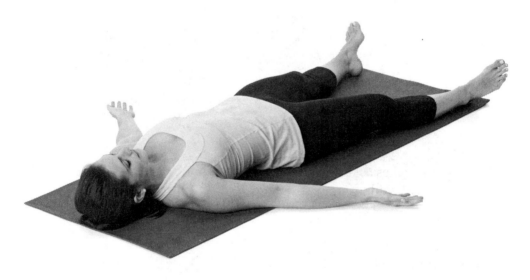

CORPSE POSE

Lie on your back with your legs extended and your arms by your sides, palms facing up. Close your eyes and breathe normally, allowing yourself to relax. Hold for 2 minutes, melting your body into the floor. Roll onto your right side and push yourself up to a seated position to end your practice.

CHAPTER 14

Daily 5-Minute Meditation

Science proves it with data: Stress-melting meditation can lower your blood pressure as much as 3 to 6 points—enough to lower risk for heart attacks and strokes. Experiencing this bliss for yourself does even more for your mind and body. Test panelists told us that the short, simple breathing exercise in this plan gave them new serenity, helped them stay on track with healthy eating and exercise, and was a use-anywhere-anytime tool for taming tension.

And it only takes 5 minutes.

Based on the widely studied, practiced, and recommended technique called mindfulness-based stress reduction, our 5-minute meditation fits into the busiest of lives. You don't need a teacher, a specific technique, or a special time or place. It just takes a few quiet minutes. Here's all you'll need to do.

1. **Find 5 minutes in the morning, afternoon, or evening that are all yours.** Shut the door and turn off your phone. Use mindfulness and the soothing rhythm of your own breath to dissolve tension.

2. **Repeat daily.** And do it more than once during the day if you'd like.

5-Minute Meditation Instructions

You will focus on your body from head to toe, breathing out tension and taking in positive vibrations. Then you'll go deeper, focusing on your breath. Here's how.

Get ready

Find a quiet area where you are not likely to be interrupted. Sit in a chair with your feet on the floor and your hips higher than your knees. You may want to sit on a cushion if you need your hips to be elevated. Your comfort is the key.

Align your head, neck, and torso so that your head is resting comfortably. Place your hands on your lap without extending your arms. Make sure your shoulders are relaxed.

Begin with calm breathing

Close your eyes and mouth, and begin to breathe through your nose slowly and smoothly, without forcing the breath. Bring the breath through your nose down into your abdomen. Let one breath flow into the next in a slow, steady rhythm.

As you exhale, release any tension, stress, worry, or fatigue that you are holding.

As you inhale, nourish your body with fresh, clean, positive energy.

Scan your body

Continue this breathing and start with the top of your head, exhaling away any tension and inhaling to nourish this area. Continue downward to your forehead, facial muscles, ears, mouth, jaw, neck, shoulders, arms, hands, and fingertips. If you feel any tightness in these areas, release it as you breathe out.

Work your way back up your arms and now down your body from your heart to your upper abdomen, lower abdomen, hips, thighs, knees, lower legs, ankles, feet, and toes. Continue to exhale away any tension that you feel in any of these areas, refreshing your body parts as you inhale.

Then work your way back up from your feet to your calves to the back of your upper legs to your lower back, midback, upper back, back of the neck, back of the head, and returning to the top of your head.

Focus on your breath

Now focus your attention on the tip of your nose between the two nostrils.

Notice the air as it exits and enters, continuing to breathe in a slow, steady rhythm. Observe the breath here for as long as you wish as you inhale and exhale. Begin counting to yourself with your next exhalation: Count 1 as you exhale, 2 as you inhale, 3 as you exhale, 4 as you inhale, 5 as you exhale. Then count back down to one: Count 5 on your next inhalation, 4 as you exhale, 3 as you inhale, 2 as you exhale, 1 as you inhale.

Continue counting your breath 1 to 5, then 5 to 1, without pausing, for as long as you'd like.

To bring yourself out of the meditation, slowly bring awareness back to your body by wiggling your hands and feet. Then gently cup your hands over your face and slowly open your eyes.

Getting the Most from Your Meditation

You may feel a little different every time you meditate, depending on the time of day and what else is happening in your life. That's fine. The idea is to be in the present, whatever the "present" is for you at that moment, and to address any stress you're feeling. There's no right way to do a breathing meditation, but it's important to feel at ease and to be gentle with yourself. The following strategies can enhance your experience.

Change positions. Instead of sitting upright in a chair, try "crocodile pose"—on your stomach, your face turned to the side on a pillow. Or try lying on your back on the floor with your legs spread slightly apart and your arms relaxed at your sides or resting gently on your stomach.

Breathe easily. There's no need to take extremely deep or long breaths. Don't hold your breath. These tips can help.

- Let the breath come naturally, at whatever pace is comfortable for you.

- Allow your inhale and exhale to flow into each other, without pause, creating a gentle rhythm.
- Remember every inhalation is nourishing and every exhalation is cleansing.
- If your thoughts wander or something distracts you, simply return your attention gently to your breath, without judging yourself.

Reflect afterward on your experience.

- How did you feel before/during/after your practice?
- Did you notice any recurring thoughts or physical sensations? Your mind and body may be telling you about an unresolved emotional issue or that another position might be more comfortable.

Be patient with yourself. Meditation is a learned skill, not magic. It takes time and practice!

Part IV

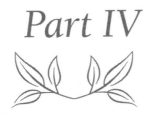

More Tools

CHAPTER 15

Alternative and Complementary Strategies for Blood Pressure

Stroll through your local pharmacy or natural foods store, surf the Internet, or switch on your TV and you're bound to come face-to-face with news, advertisements, and come-ons for "alternative" high blood pressure remedies. Figuring out which ones may be worth adding to your pressure-control arsenal—and which ones should be avoided—can be a real challenge. We're here to help. We've combed through hundreds of research studies to sort out the truth about 20 widely used alternative approaches.

The bottom line? No alternative remedy is a magic bullet that can take the place of a healthy diet, regular exercise, and stress-soothing relaxation (and medication if you need it). A few strategies could be smart add-ons, while many others are duds, and some could be downright dangerous. Here's what you need to know.

Meditation

A short daily meditation focused on your breath is a component of the Lower Your Blood Pressure Naturally plan. Plenty of research suggests that several styles of formal meditation yield important pressure-lowering benefits. Here are the details.

Transcendental Meditation (TM)

This technique uses a repeated word or phrase, called a mantra, to help you leave wandering, worrying thoughts behind and experience pure awareness. It is the best-studied type of meditation for lowering blood pressure. In studies of a wide range of people—including Caucasians, African Americans, teens, middle-agers, and the elderly—a regular TM practice lowered systolic blood pressure an average of 4.7 points and diastolic blood pressure by 3.2 points, enough to reduce risk for heart attacks and strokes.[1]

Mindfulness-Based Stress Reduction (MBSR)

Similar to the meditation you'll find in this plan, MBSR involves using breathing and body awareness to increase mindfulness for better coping and to bring more comfort to your daily life. Used to ease tension, it is emerging as a potent way to turn down the fight-or-flight response that contributes to high blood pressure. In a small 2012 study from Johns Hopkins Bloomberg School of Public Health of 20 older adults with high blood pressure, those who practiced MBSR once a week for 8 weeks saw a 21-point drop in systolic blood pressure and a 16-point drop in diastolic pressure.[2] In other research from Duke University, the University of Calgary, and the Tom Baker Cancer Centre in Alberta, Canada, MBSR has also reduced BP in people with diabetes[3] and with breast[4] or prostate cancer.[5]

Zen Meditation

This Buddhist practice involves letting go of thoughts to find your "true mind." And it lowered diastolic pressure 6 points, according to a 2013 American Heart Association review of alternative and complementary therapies for hypertension.[6]

How It May Help

All forms of meditation can lower levels of the stress hormones cortisol, epinephrine, and norepinephrine in your bloodstream. These boost blood pressure by tightening arteries; having less of them on hand encourages blood vessels to relax.

In addition, meditation seems to lower levels of aldosterone, a hormone that raises blood pressure by encouraging the kidneys to absorb more sodium and water. Reducing aldosterone can reduce the amount of excess fluid in your blood, which in turn lowers BP, explain researchers from Georgia Health Sciences University, now Georgia Regents University.[7] Meditation may also help indirectly by reducing stress, making it easier to stick with healthy habits, like quitting smoking, they say.

Should You Try It?

Practicing some form of stress-reducing meditation regularly is a smart, effective add-on strategy for better blood pressure. Start with the 5-minute meditation in this plan, and then investigate more formal techniques if you're interested.

Tai Chi

This slow, dancelike, total-body exercise is a moving meditation that can calm blood pressure almost as much as a regular, moderate-intensity cardio routine, say Johns Hopkins University researchers. In one older yet notable study of 62 people with hypertension, those who did a 30-minute tai chi routine four times a week for 12 weeks reduced blood pressure by 7 points, a result that surprised researchers.[8] And in a review of 26 published studies examining the effectiveness of tai chi for reducing high blood pressure, 85 percent of the studies demonstrated a reduction in blood pressure.[9]

How It May Help

Tai chi combines deep diaphragmatic breathing with continuous body motions, a mix that might help lower blood pressure by relieving stress and working muscles.

Should You Try It?

Other cardiovascular activities have a bigger effect on blood pressure. Still, tai chi is a good add-on strategy for keeping pressure lower. It is a great alternative to cardio exercise if you absolutely hate to sweat or have limitations that make low-impact, gentler movements a better choice for you.

Biofeedback

Biofeedback is a technique that uses electronic devices to give you information about various bodily functions, such as breathing and heart rate. The feedback provided helps you make changes that will allow you to relax more fully.

One biofeedback breathing device, called Resperate, plays musical notes and melodies that help you slow down your breathing. Does biofeedback really help lower BP? British scientists who reviewed 36 biofeedback studies for a 2010 report say no.[10] But when the American Heart Association reviewed 13 studies of Resperate, the group found that regular use lowered BP by 3 to 4 points.

How It May Help

Resperate uses tones and melodies to slow and synchronize breathing. This can evoke the body's relaxation response, which can activate the parasympathetic nervous system to calm blood pressure.

Should You Try It?

Maybe, as an add-on therapy, if you have the time and the money. The device costs about $200, and the maker recommends using it for 15 minutes three to four times a week.[11] One caveat: A lingering concern is that favorable studies of this device were all sponsored by the manufacturer, say Oxford University researchers who reviewed eight Resperate studies in 2012.[12]

Acupuncture

In acupuncture, a trained practitioner inserts thin needles at various points on the body to stimulate the flow of energy, called chi. This ancient component of traditional Chinese medicine has some modern science behind it, suggesting that it may help lower blood pressure.

In 1996 the World Health Organization said it was an option for early, mild hypertension. And some well-designed studies have found benefits. In one Korean study of people already using medications and/or lifestyle strategies to lower BP, acupuncture reduced their numbers by an additional 7 to 14 points.

Not all research has been positive, though. In a large American study called SHARP (short for Stop Hypertension with the Acupuncture Research Program), 192 people with hypertension received real or "fake" acupuncture. Both groups saw BP fall 2 to 4 points.[13]

How It May Help

Some research suggests acupuncture might soothe blood pressure by calming the body's fight-or-flight response and by cooling off inflammation, which can damage and tighten arteries.

Should You Try It?

Maybe, as an add-on therapy. If it helps, it's not clear how often you'll need follow-up visits to keep the benefits going.[14]

Massage

Could getting the kinks and tight spots worked out of your muscles have a blood pressure–lowering benefit? Maybe. In an interesting study from Iran, women with prehypertension who got a Swedish massage three times a week for 10 weeks lowered their systolic pressure levels by 12 points. Pressure stayed lower for 3 days after a massage, but long-term effects weren't checked.[15]

How It May Help

Researchers aren't sure how a muscle-melting rubdown helps BP, but it could be by reducing stress.

Should You Try It?

We don't see this as an ongoing strategy for blood pressure control. But it's nice to know that if you are feeling extra-stressed or want to give yourself a relaxing treat, massage not only feels good but may temporarily lower blood pressure.

Laughter

Seriously! A Japanese study involving 79 people with high blood pressure found that giggles and guffaws reduced BP numbers. Thirty study volunteers did "laughter yoga," breathing exercises combined with laughter stimulated by playful eye contact with class leaders. They also watched a comedy performance. Blood pressure was 7 points lower right after laughter sessions, compared to people in a control group who didn't get the chance to yuck it up. In a 2008 study, presented at a meeting of the American Society of Hypertension,[16] alternating laughter and deep breathing for 20 to 30 minutes several times over 3 weeks lowered blood pressure.[17]

How It May Help

Laughter may help by releasing feel-good brain chemicals and reducing production of stress hormones. The laughter–healthier heart connection has gotten attention from several researchers. In one study from California's Loma Linda University of 48 heart attack survivors, those who got a daily half-hour dose of humor for 1 year had lower blood pressure, fewer off-beat heart rhythms, lower levels of stress hormones, and 80 percent fewer repeat heart attacks.[18]

Should You Try It?

This is a great reason to laugh more often, but it's not a substitute for other blood pressure–lowering steps. When you're looking for something to do on a Friday night, watch a funny movie or TV show or visit a comedy club. Tell more jokes, read the comics in the newspaper, and check out books by your favorite funny writers from the library.

Music

In the same Japanese study that measured the effects of laughter, another 32 people with high blood pressure got a 6-point BP drop by enjoying music more often. For 3 months, they sang, listened to their favorite songs, and did stretching exercises along to music daily.[19]

How It May Help

As with laughter, music may help by reducing levels of stress hormones. Listening to calming music nudges you to breathe more slowly, which helps dilate arteries and decrease blood pressure.

Should You Try It?

Don't give up other BP-lowering strategies in favor of listening to your favorite Justin Timberlake songs, but do make time for the music you love. Sing in the shower or in your car, join a choir, spin the radio dial from news to music more often. These everyday choices can affect your physiology in ways that promote healthier blood pressure levels. Your favorite music—be it calming or more upbeat—is also a great addition to the yoga routines you will do on the Lower Your Blood Pressure Naturally plan.

Vitamin D

Could this so-called sunshine vitamin reach into your circulatory system to calm high BP? In a 2013 study from Boston's Brigham and Women's Hospital of 250 African American women and men with hypertension, researchers found that those who took a daily D supplement reduced their numbers. Getting 1,000 IUs per day lowered systolic blood pressure (the top number) 7 points. The results are significant for African Americans, who are at higher risk for high blood pressure and have lower blood levels of D compared to the US population as a whole. The researchers say the findings may also be important for others, as many Americans are low in D.

And in a 2009 University of Wisconsin study of 1,334 Hispanic and African American women and men, those with low blood levels of D were more likely to have high blood pressure than those with healthy levels.[20] The researchers note that bringing low D levels up could reduce blood pressure by 1.5 to 2.3 points, enough to reduce risk for heart disease–related deaths by a whopping 10 to 15 percent. Low levels of D may contribute to weight gain, which raises blood pressure, the University of Wisconsin researchers add.

How It May Help

Researchers aren't sure how D might help lower blood pressure. Experts think it may have a beneficial effect on kidney function by helping to keep levels of the pressure-raising parathyroid hormone in check.

Should You Try It?

Vitamin D alone cannot control high blood pressure. And it doesn't seem to help a type called isolated systolic hypertension, in which just the top number is elevated, says a 2013 study from Scotland's University of Dundee.[21] The Institute of Medicine recommends getting 600 to 800 IUs of vitamin D per day. The safe upper limit is 2,000 IUs per day, but it's wise to ask your doctor about a blood test for D first. If your levels are low, your doctor may prescribe a higher dose for several weeks or more, and then recheck your levels.[22]

Coenzyme Q10

A vitamin-like substance produced naturally in the human body, CoQ10 helps mitochondria—the tiny power plants in your cells—function optimally. People with heart disease and other conditions have been found to have low levels. CoQ10 levels also decline naturally with age. Research suggests that supplements might help reduce blood pressure levels.

In one 8-week study of 59 men already taking medication for high blood pressure, daily CoQ10 reduced blood pressure by about 9 percent, report researchers from India's NKP Salve Institute of Medical Science.[23] A 12-week study—which was conducted by researchers from the Department of Veterans Affairs Medical Center in Boise, Idaho—of 83 people with isolated systolic hypertension found that 60 milligrams a day got similar results.[24] In an Australian study of 74 people with diabetes and hypertension, 100 milligrams of CoQ10 twice daily significantly reduced blood pressure in 12 weeks.[25]

How It May Help

CoQ10 may lower BP by mopping up cell-damaging oxygen molecules called free radicals before they can ding your arteries.

Should You Try It?

Don't use CoQ10 or any supplement instead of lifestyle steps proven to tame high blood pressure. At best, it's an add-on. The *Natural Medicines Comprehensive Database* rates CoQ10 as "possibly effective" for high blood pressure.[26] The National Library of Medicine says this supplement is "likely safe" when taken for high blood pressure in two daily doses of 60 to 100 milligrams.

It may be of special interest for people who also take cholesterol-lowering statin drugs, which can reduce CoQ10 levels in the body, report researchers from the Cleveland Clinic who reviewed the supplement's potential benefits for statin users with hypertension. But, they note, its side effects can include nausea, vomiting, diarrhea, and anorexia as well as allergic rashes and headaches. And it can interact with anticlotting medicines, such as warfarin, aspirin, and clopidogrel (Plavix).[27]

Fish Oil

Does it help, or doesn't it? Some studies report that EPA and DHA—the two omega-3 fatty acids found in fatty fish and in fish oil capsules—may reduce blood pressure in people with mild hypertension. However, other studies have had conflicting results. In 2013, researchers from the UK's University of Sheffield sorted out the fish oil–BP debate when they reviewed 17 fish oil studies involving 1,524 people.

The verdict: It may help people with hypertension reduce their numbers by 1.47 to 2.56 points. But fish oil didn't reduce the blood pressure of people who did not have hypertension.

Blood Pressure Supplements: Not Ready for Prime Time!

Pricey pills and capsules with names that seem to promise better blood pressure control line the shelves of supermarkets, drugstores, and health food stores. You'll also find them online. And studies continue to pop up in the media suggesting that others could help. Some show promise, but more research is needed. Our advice: Never take any supplement in place of prescribed blood pressure drugs or instead of making healthy changes proven to help BP! And think twice about the following widely touted supplements that research shows aren't ready for prime time.

GLUCOMANNAN: Made from the root of the Japanese konjac tree, this fiber supplement has a growing reputation as a weight loss aid. You'll find Web sites claiming it helps with high BP, too. But a 2008 University of Connecticut review concluded that it doesn't reduce blood pressure.[28]

YARROW: *Achillea wilhelmsii* and other types of yarrow are touted online for lowering blood pressure, but evidence comes only from a few small, poorly designed studies.[29]

GREEN COFFEE BEAN EXTRACT: A 2005 study from Japan suggests that this extract may reduce blood pressure in people with mild hypertension. But it was performed by a consumer products company, not impartial researchers. And New York University experts note that the study's design might have exaggerated the benefits.[30]

PYCNOGENOL: The well-regarded *Natural Medicines Comprehensive Database* rates this pine bark extract as "possibly effective" for lowering systolic blood pressure.[31] In one University of Arizona study of people with diabetes and mild to moderate hypertension, those who took pycnogenol for 12 weeks saw their numbers decline somewhat. While possibly safe to use for up to 6 months, pycnogenol can cause dizziness, gut problems, headaches, and mouth ulcers. It can also increase immune system activity, which makes it off-limits for people with autoimmune conditions—like multiple sclerosis, lupus, and rheumatoid arthritis—and for people taking drugs that decrease immune system activity—including corticosteroids, oral and topical tacrolimus (an eczema drug), and cyclosporine (for dry eyes)—and drugs to prevent organ transplant rejection, such as sirolimus, daclizumab, and azathioprine.

PSYLLIUM: "Blond psyllium" is garnering a reputation as a natural blood pressure treatment. In fact, it's the same as the psyllium fiber found in drugstore supplements designed to improve regularity and help control cholesterol levels.[32] Evidence comes from studies that compared diets with psyllium supplementation to low-fiber diets, and the BP benefits likely come from the extra fiber, not from special properties of the psyllium. In a 12-week study involving overweight people, those who ate a diet packed with high-fiber foods reduced their blood pressure numbers, whereas those who got psyllium supplements did not.[33]

DIMETHYL SULFOXIDE (DMSO): An industrial solvent, DMSO is a by-product of making paper that is also sometimes used in medical studies to help dissolve drugs or other chemicals. Promoted as an alternative cancer treatment since the 1960s,[34] it is also gaining a folk reputation for treating high blood pressure. But steer clear. In the United States, pharmaceutical-quality DMSO is FDA-approved as a specialized drug treatment for a bladder condition called interstitial cystitis (it's inserted into the bladder via a catheter). It has been studied as an injected drug to lower dangerous high blood pressure in the brain, but there's no evidence that the supplements lower blood pressure.

Health experts warn consumers against using DMSO supplements, creams, and ointments on their own. "It is not approved for over-the-counter use in any form due to inadequate evidences of efficacy and potential toxicities," note alternative medicine experts at New York's Memorial Sloan Kettering Cancer Center.[35] Some nonprescription DMSO products might be "industrial grade" and are not intended for human use. They can contain impurities that can affect health: Strong allergic reactions, vision problems, and dangerous interactions with blood thinners and heart medications have been reported.

RESVERATROL: If you're a lab mouse, resveratrol—a cell-protecting polyphenol found naturally in grapes, wine, and grape juice—might lower your risk for high blood pressure, says a 2013 study from Canada's University of Alberta.[36] But human beings may be wasting their money on this popular supplement, touted for everything from weight loss to protection against heart disease and Alzheimer's disease. Your best bet: Enjoy resveratrol when you munch a handful of grapes or sip a glass of grape juice or wine.

How It May Help

The omega-3 fatty acids in fish oil may keep arteries flexible.

Should You Try It?

Getting omega-3s from fish and from plant sources (walnuts, flaxseed, canola oil) is a heart-smart strategy. If you have heart disease, add 1,000 milligrams of omega-3s daily from a supplement. Don't take more than 3,000 milligrams a day without talking to your doctor. Too much can boost bleeding risk.[37]

Pomegranate Juice

Sipping 17 ounces of this beverage a day lowered blood pressure by about 5 points in a 2011 study from the UK's Queen Margaret University. The report made headlines, but you may not have heard about the drawbacks. The study was small (just 20 volunteers), funded by a food maker, and presented at a conference (not published in a scientific journal). And those 17 ounces of juice contain a whopping 255 calories!

How It May Help

Pomegranate juice is a great source of potassium. Seventeen ounces contains about 1,133 milligrams of this pressure-lowering mineral—almost one-fourth of the amount you need every day. It also contains polyphenols that ramp up your body's antioxidant system to protect arteries and keep them flexible.[38]

Should You Try It?

Enjoy a glass now and then if you like pomegranate juice, but don't depend on it as a daily pressure-lowering measure. It's tough remembering to drink two glasses per day. And there's scant evidence that pomegranate extracts influence blood pressure.[39] Bottom line? The National Library of Medicine notes that "there isn't enough information to know if drinking pomegranate juice helps to prevent heart disease–related events such as heart attack."[40]

CHAPTER 16

Total Cardiovascular Health: Beyond High Blood Pressure

You're reading this book because you or someone you love has high blood pressure or is at high risk for it. You want better numbers, but you really want much, much more. Your true hope (and ours) is that you'll sidestep high blood pressure's toll–the heart disease, heart attacks, strokes, heart failure, and other pressure-related health problems that can alter your life or even cut it short.

It's an intelligent desire. Cardiovascular disease, the health condition that includes heart problems and blood vessel trouble, kills 386,436 men and 401,495 women a year, according to the American Heart Association (more than cancer, Alzheimer's disease, and accidents combined).[1] Heart disease, stroke, and high blood pressure are among the 15 top reasons that 45 million Americans are disabled, the association says.

Nurturing a healthy heart and healthy arteries means taking care of your blood pressure as well as your cholesterol levels, triglycerides, and blood sugar. Working with your doctor and following this plan can help with all of these. As you'll discover in this chapter, the eating, exercise, and stress-reducing strategies you'll deploy on the Lower Your Blood Pressure

Naturally plan also have the power to help rebalance blood fats and help keep blood sugar in check.

Plenty of us can benefit. Sixty-four percent of people with hypertension also have high cholesterol levels, says a 2013 analysis of national health data by the University of South Carolina.[2] And three out of four people with diabetes also have hypertension. Overall, one in eight adults in the United States have two of these three conditions—high BP, high cholesterol, or diabetes—according to the Centers for Disease Control and Prevention. One in 33 have all three. But the true numbers may be even higher. In fact, 8 percent of adults in the United States have undiagnosed high blood pressure, another 8 percent have undiagnosed high cholesterol, and 3 percent have diabetes but don't know it.[3]

Another 1 in 10 Americans have prehypertension plus prediabetes. Individually, higher-than-healthy blood pressure and elevated blood sugar numbers threaten your heart, but put them together and this duo becomes an even more potent menace due, in part, to high levels of body-wide inflammation, say Louisiana State University researchers in a study presented at the 2010 meeting of the American Society of Hypertension.

Your best move? Know your numbers and take action. Reducing high cholesterol and high blood pressure can slash your risk for heart disease by more than 50 percent, report University of South Carolina researchers in a headline-grabbing 2013 study.[4] If you have diabetes plus high blood pressure, controlling your blood sugar and reducing your blood pressure by 10 points can lower your risk for a heart attack by 11 percent.[5]

The destiny of your heart and arteries is in your hands. When Northwestern University researchers tracked the heart health of thousands of families for three generations for a 2010 study, they found that only a small percentage of heart risk was passed genetically from generation to generation. Most risk was due to lifestyle choices. In fact, another large study called INTERHEART found that 90 percent is due to lifestyle choices. You've got the power to keep your heart healthy. Here's what you need to know.

Cholesterol and Triglycerides: Aim for a Better Balance

Cholesterol itself isn't a bad thing. Your body uses this waxy fat—made from the cholesterol and saturated fat in the food you eat—to manufacture coatings for your cells, bile acid for digestion, and essential sex hormones, like estrogen and testosterone.

The trouble comes when there's too much bad cholesterol, or too little of the good stuff, in your bloodstream. Down too many ice cream bars, grilled cheese sandwiches, or fried chicken—all major sources of saturated fat—and levels of "lousy" LDL cholesterol soar. Avoid exercise and skimp on good fats and levels of "helpful" HDL cholesterol can fall.

The combo is bad news for your arteries. LDLs, the villain in every magazine ad and TV commercial for cholesterol-lowering drugs, burrow into artery walls. This may happen simply because there are too many and they oversaturate artery linings or because LDL cholesterol becomes dense when it gets oxidized in your bloodstream by rogue oxygen molecules called free radicals. Either way, when the LDLs enter the lining of arteries, they attract the attention of immune system warriors called macrophages. Together, the macrophages and LDLs form pools of foamy, gunky plaque. These deposits can cause blockages, or they can burst, creating blood clots that trigger heart attacks and strokes.

Meanwhile, HDLs are your bloodstream's cholesterol waste-disposal trucks, hauling LDLs off to your liver for removal. Low HDLs also boost odds for heart disease and strokes.

What about triglycerides? These fat particles contain the calories your body couldn't burn immediately after a meal. Packaged into little blobs, they're in your bloodstream because they're en route to your fat cells for storage. Too many also boost risk for heart disease.

One in three Americans has high LDLs,[6] one in four has low HDLs, and one in three has high triglycerides.[7] In women, high triglycerides increase the risk of heart disease more than they do in men. For those people who are carbohydrate sensitive or have prediabetes or diabetes, triglycerides are often high. They can be decreased with dietary changes.

What happens when you have high blood pressure plus off-balance cholesterol levels: High-force blood rips tiny tears in artery walls that let cholesterol in. Constricted arteries, often a feature of high blood pressure, can contribute to blockages caused by bulging plaque. And by pummeling arteries, high blood pressure can also rip plaque deposits open, leading to the formation of dangerous blood clots that cause heart attacks and strokes.

Total heart (and brain) health solution: Clearly, you need low LDLs and high HDLs along with healthy BP to stop this scenario. Lowering your LDLs 40 points can reduce your risk for a heart attack by 23 percent and for a stroke by 17 percent.[8] At the same time, a 1-point increase in your HDLs can lower heart disease risk as much as 6 percent. (In women, increasing HDLs has a greater protective effect than in men. Increasing HDLs in men can decrease the risk of heart disease by 2 to 3 percent, but in women it is as much as 7 percent.)[9] Here's how to find out where you stand, what to do next, and how the Lower Your Blood Pressure Naturally plan can help you rebalance your blood fats.

Testing and Numbers

The American Heart Association recommends that everyone age 20 and older have a fasting blood test of their cholesterol and triglyceride levels every 5 years. But talk to your doctor; you may need more frequent checks if you have high blood pressure or other heart disease risk factors, are over age 45 for men or 50 for women, or have total cholesterol over 200 or HDL cholesterol under 40. (If you have a family history of either high cholesterol or heart disease, screenings may begin earlier and be done more regularly.)

Before your test, fast for 9 to 12 hours, skipping food and beverages. (Ask your doctor what to do about any medications you take regularly.) A blood sample will be drawn and sent to a lab for analysis. Although this is traditionally a fasting test, sometimes your doctor might suggest you have something to eat prior to the test. There's some evidence that a nonfasting check could provide important information about insulin resistance, another heart disease risk factor.

Don't know your numbers or what they should be? You're not alone. In one national survey of 1,008 women, just 21 percent knew what the best LDL number was for them and just 37 percent knew what a healthy HDL level should be.[10] In another study, women who did not know their cholesterol levels had an 88 percent higher risk for heart disease than those who did.[11] Guys face a similar knowledge gap: Just 65 percent have had a cholesterol check in the past 5 years. Men are more likely than women to have high LDLs and low HDLs, and they're less likely to get treatment or work with a doctor to hit a healthier balance.[12, 13, 14] Wondering about your results? Here's what they mean and what to aim for.

Total Cholesterol: Aim for 199 mg/dL or lower

Total cholesterol adds together HDLs, LDLs, and a few other blood fats.

- Less than 200 mg/dL: Optimal
- 200 to 239 mg/dL: Borderline high
- 240 mg/dL and above: High

HDLs: Aim for 50 mg/dL or higher for women, 40 mg/dL or higher for men

- Less than 50 mg/dL (for women)/less than 40 mg/dL (for men): Low
- 60 mg/dL and above: High (which is protective against heart disease)

LDLs: Aim for 99 mg/dL or lower

- Less than 100 mg/dL: Optimal (aim for 70 mg/dL or lower if you have diabetes or heart disease)
- 100 to 129 mg/dL: Near or just above optimal
- 130 to 159 mg/dL: Borderline high
- 160 to 189 mg/dL: High
- 190 mg/dL and above: Very high

Triglycerides: Aim for 99 mg/dL or lower

These blood fats can rise if you are overweight, inactive, smoke, or overindulge in alcohol or if you eat a diet that's too high in carbohydrates.

- Less than 100 mg/dL: Optimal
- 100 to 149 mg/dL: Normal
- 150 to 199 mg/dL: Borderline high
- 200 to 499 mg/dL: High
- 500 mg/dL and above: Very high

High HDLs Don't "Erase" High LDLs

Got high levels of good-for-you HDL cholesterol? Give yourself a pat on the back, but don't rest yet. Heart experts want you to know that while high HDLs do protect your heart and arteries by whisking more "lousy" LDL cholesterol out of circulation, they can't wipe out the heart risk posed by high levels of LDLs. Science is just beginning to understand that not all types of HDLs are equally protective and that some LDLs are more dense and more atherogenic than others. Your best bet for a healthy ticker: Keep HDLs up and LDLs down.[15]

Five Steps to Better Blood Fats

These top lifestyle moves can help get your numbers back within a healthy range. Your doctor may also recommend cholesterol-lowering drugs. The good news: Many elements of the Lower Your Blood Pressure Naturally plan can help you attain and sustain healthier cholesterol and triglyceride levels.

1. **Lose weight.** Plenty of research shows that weight loss helps trim high LDLs by as much as 22 percent.[16]

2. **Exercise.** It's great for reducing LDLs and raising HDLs, and the routines in this plan are proven to help. Norwegian researchers report that interval training—as you do on the plan—does more to boost HDLs than steady-paced exercise.[17] In one West Virginia University School of Medicine study, people who lifted weights for just 4 weeks saw an average 5 percent drop in LDL cholesterol.[18]

3. **Slash "bad fats," boost "good fats."** Cutting out trans fats and keeping your intake of saturated fats low are two important ways to tamp down high LDLs. The avocado, nuts, and olive oil you'll enjoy on this plan are building blocks for heart-healthy HDLs. And by slashing saturated fats (found in full-fat dairy products, fatty cuts of meat, poultry skin, and many processed foods) and eliminating trans fats (found in many packaged and processed foods), the plan removes a big source of "raw materials" for excess LDLs.

4. **Eat more soluble fiber.** It's found in many whole grains, fruits, vegetables, and beans, which are plentiful in the eating plan. Soluble fiber reduces LDLs two ways: It reduces the absorption of cholesterol from the food you eat, and it forms a gel in your digestive system that traps cholesterol-rich bile acids, whisking them out of your body; as a result, your liver pulls more cholesterol from your bloodstream to make more bile acids.

5. **Ease stress.** Chronic stress can raise LDLs, perhaps by raising levels of body-wide inflammation or by prompting the liver to send out more fats that your body can use as fuel when the primitive fight-or-flight response is activated, say British researchers.[19] Easing tension shuts down this process and may also boost levels of good HDLs, Stanford University heart health experts say.[20]

Prediabetes and Diabetes: Get Serious about Blood Sugar

Diabetes and prediabetes can wreak life-threatening, body-wide havoc. High blood sugar doubles or even quadruples risk for heart attacks and strokes. And it also increases your risk for kidney problems, vision loss, nerve damage, and even lower-leg amputations and dementia. Other risks include higher odds for 24 types of cancer (including those of the pancreas, liver, kidneys, and thyroid) and a 70 percent higher risk for bone fractures.

But diabetes, which affects 25.8 million Americans,[21] carries another heart risk. One in four people with high blood sugar also cope with depression, perhaps due to increased levels of body-wide inflammation. This directly increases heart risks, but as you can imagine, depression also threatens your overall health simply by zapping the energy and confidence you need to make healthy choices every day. No wonder a 2011 study from Harvard Medical School found that diabetes plus depression raised a woman's odds for fatal heart disease fivefold.[22]

Risk rises even before your blood sugar hits the diabetic range. Prediabetes is the higher-than-healthy blood sugar, due to an insulin resistance, that affects 79 million Americans,[23] and it increases the odds for heart attack, stroke,[24] dementia,[25] early damage to eyes[26] and kidneys,[27] and leg pain due to circulation problems.[28] Prediabetes is also associated with increased belly fat, which compounds your risk of developing hypertension.

What happens when you have diabetes plus high blood pressure? Three-quarters of the people with diabetes face this problem. The combination turns heart disease, stroke, and other circulation problems into major health risks. In 2002, diabetes became a coronary artery disease risk equivalent, and more than 50 percent of people with diabetes will have heart disease, making it the greatest risk for those with diabetes. If you have diabetes, all of your heart disease risk factors should be screened carefully and be well managed to prevent the development of heart disease.

Testing and Numbers

The American Diabetes Association recommends regular checks starting at age 45, but you may need to start sooner or be checked more frequently if you are overweight; are physically active less than three times a week; have a parent or sibling with diabetes; are of African American, Hispanic/Latino, American Indian, Asian American, or Pacific Islander descent; had pregnancy (gestational) diabetes; or gave birth to a baby weighing 9 pounds or more.[29] Make an appointment with your doctor (or check with a local walk-in clinic, as many offer diabetes screenings).

Two blood tests are widely used to screen for diabetes. If your doctor suspects a problem, you may be asked to return for a recheck before a diagnosis is given. Here are the details.

A1c test

This test measures your average blood glucose for the past 2 to 3 months. You won't have to fast before taking it, and the results may be available in minutes. Following are the results and what they mean.

- 5.6 percent or lower: Normal
- 5.7 to 6.4 percent: Prediabetes
- 6.5 percent or higher: Diabetes

Fasting plasma glucose

This test checks your fasting blood glucose levels. It's usually performed in the morning after a fast with nothing to eat or drink (except water) for at least 8 hours beforehand. Following are the results and what they mean.

Other Blood Sugar Tests

Occasionally, doctors check blood sugar in two other ways.

A random or "casual" plasma glucose test is done without fasting. Your doctor may use this check if you're having severe symptoms, such as blurry vision or unexplained weight loss, that could be caused by extremely high blood sugar levels or undiagnosed diabetes. You may have diabetes if your test result is 200 mg/dL or higher.

An oral glucose tolerance test (OGTT) shows how your body processes blood sugar right after a meal. It can detect early blood sugar problems that may not show up on an A1c or fasting check. For this test, you drink a specially formulated sweet beverage. Your blood sugar is checked beforehand and then 2 hours later. You may have prediabetes if your blood sugar is 140 mg/dL to 199 mg/dL and diabetes if your blood sugar is 200 mg/dL or higher. A version of the OGTT is given to women during pregnancy to detect gestational diabetes. You may have it if your fasting blood sugar is 95 mg/dL or higher or if your blood sugar is 180 mg/dL 1 hour after having the special drink, 155 mg/dL or higher 2 hours afterward, or 140 mg/dL or higher at 3 hours.

- Under 100 mg/dL: Normal
- 100 to 125 mg/dL: Prediabetes
- 126 mg/dL and higher: Diabetes

Six Steps That Control Blood Sugar

Knowing your blood sugar level and working with your doctor if you already have diabetes or prediabetes are crucial. You may be prescribed blood sugar–lowering medications for diabetes. These lifestyle strategies can help.

1. **Lose a little weight.** Losing just 7 percent of your body weight can reduce your risk for moving from prediabetes to diabetes by an impressive 58 percent, research shows. Dropping excess pounds and trimming belly fat can also help you gain better control of

Bean Bonus for People with Diabetes

Bursting with blood sugar–friendly soluble fiber, dried beans can improve diabetes control while lowering heart disease risk, according to a 2012 study from St. Michael's Hospital in Toronto. People with high blood sugar who ate a bean-rich diet for 3 months lowered their A1c (a measure of long-term blood sugar control) by a significant 0.5 percent. Their systolic blood pressure (the top number in a BP reading) fell 4.5 points, too.[30] You'll find plenty of beans to enjoy on this plan. Creamy white beans are incorporated into side dishes, entrées, and a delicious soup in Phase 1, and black beans and kidney beans star in breakfast tostadas, lunchtime salads, and delicious burgers.

diabetes by making your cells more sensitive to the hormone that regulates blood sugar absorption.

2. **Eat fewer refined carbs and more fiber-rich produce.** Sweets, sugary drinks, and foods made with white flour can boost blood sugar higher, faster after a meal. Avoid the spikes by enjoying plenty of fiber- and nutrient-rich vegetables and fruits. The fiber helps you stay full (a weight loss aid) and slows the rise in blood sugar after a meal. Be sure to include greens: People who ate the most reduced their diabetes risk 14 percent in one Harvard study. Why? Greens are rich in magnesium, a Power Mineral that helps regulate blood sugar (as well as blood pressure).[31]

3. **Choose whole grains.** Three to five daily servings of whole grains reduced diabetes risk 26 percent in a 2012 University of California, Los Angeles, study.[32] Including whole grains in your diet if you already have diabetes can keep blood sugar lower and steadier after meals, too.[33] In 2010, researchers from the Cooper Institute in Dallas reported that people who followed an eating plan packed with produce, whole grains, and lean protein were 13 to 28 percent less likely to have metabolic syndrome, a prediabetic condition that boosts risk for diabetes and heart disease.

Why Your Arteries and Blood Sugar Love a Good Night's Sleep

Shortchanging yourself on sleep—whether you were up late working, watching late-night TV, or tossing and turning with insomnia—boosts risk for diabetes by 24 percent[34] and increases your odds for a fatal heart attack by up to 22 percent, as much as smoking.

Good sleep can help you maintain great blood pressure levels. The rest of this bedtime story's happy ending? Plenty of deep, restorative slumber helps your blood sugar and your heart, too.

The diabetes connection: Short sleep reduces insulin sensitivity, your body's ability to obey commands from the hormone insulin to absorb blood sugar, a key metabolic problem in diabetes.[35] Disrupted sleep can make controlling your blood sugar more challenging,[36] according to the Joslin Diabetes Center. And insomnia ups insulin resistance in people with diabetes.[37]

The heart connection: In a 2013 study from the National Institute for Public Health and the Environment in the Netherlands, sleep increased the effectiveness of heart-pampering strategies, like eating a healthy diet, exercising, not smoking, and drinking alcohol in moderation. Practicing just those four reduced risk for a heart attack by 57 percent and for a fatal attack by 67 percent. Adding good sleep boosted protection to 65 percent and 83 percent, respectively.[38] In contrast, regularly sleeping less than 6 hours per night could raise your heart attack risk fivefold over time, Japanese researchers report. The reason? Researchers aren't sure, but they do know that deep sleep repairs tissues and resets important regulatory systems throughout your body.

Obstructive sleep apnea (OSA), meanwhile, increases heart attack risk by 30 percent.[39] And up to 23 percent of people with diabetes have OSA.[40] If you have OSA, loose tissue in your throat blocks your airways repeatedly during sleep, leading to loud snoring, gasping, and breaks in breathing that disrupt sleep and reduce oxygen levels in your blood.

What you can do: Get a better night's sleep, and get help for sleep apnea (see "Is High Blood Pressure Keeping You Awake?" on page 25).

Seven Surprising Facts about Smoking and Heart Health

Smoking is on the decline in America. But if you're among the one in five men or one in six women who's still lighting up, we've got some compelling reasons for you to make plans to quit.

- Smoking one pack a day raises your risk for type 2 diabetes by 70 percent.[41]

- Social smoking is still dangerous. Smoking just one to four cigarettes a day triples your risk for heart disease.

- Light smoking is also dangerous. Puffing four to seven cigarettes a day causes only 30 percent less harm to your arteries than smoking 23 cigarettes a day.[42]

- The 7,000 chemicals in cigarette smoke include 69 known cancer-causing compounds as well as nicotine, carbon monoxide, and oxidant gases that deplete your body's supply of health-protecting antioxidants and boost the size of your red blood cells, making them more likely to form heart- and brain-threatening clots.[43]

- Metals in cigarette smoke—aluminum, cadmium, copper, lead, mercury, nickel, and zinc—can damage and destroy blood vessel linings, making it easier for plaque to load up in artery walls.

- Ten minutes after your first cigarette of the day, levels of the stress hormone epinephrine jump 150 percent, making your heart work harder.

- Smoking is responsible for one in three heart and blood vessel disease deaths in the United States.[44]

4. **Eat less saturated fat and more good fats.** Saturated fat reduces your body's ability to obey commands from insulin, the hormone that tells cells to mop up blood sugar. In contrast, monounsaturated fats—found in nuts, avocados, and olive oil—can help prevent this insulin resistance.[45]

5. **Move!** Exercise prompts your muscles to sip more sugar directly from your bloodstream even if you're insulin resistant, automatically lowering blood sugar. At the same time, it helps your body regain insulin sensitivity in the long run and can help you lose weight and belly fat, too. The interval walks and strength training you'll do on this plan are proven to help improve insulin sensitivity faster.[46, 47] Exercise also dilates your arteries and turns on your parasympathetic nervous system, both of which keep your blood pressure lower.

6. **Relax.** Taking time every day to reduce stress, as you will with the daily meditation on this plan, is a proven way to gain better blood sugar control without increasing medication. In one study, people who practiced mindfulness-based stress reduction (a form of meditation) lowered their A1c levels by 0.5 percent, a significant drop.[48]

Multitasking Lifestyle Steps Cut Cancer Risk, Too

Pampering your heart slashes your risk for cancer, according to a Northwestern University study. Researchers compared the health of 13,360 women and men and found that those who practiced six or seven key heart-protecting strategies lowered cancer risk 51 percent. Maintaining four cut risk 33 percent, and keeping up with just one strategy reduced risk 21 percent. The important steps? They're the same ones you'll make while following the Lower Your Blood Pressure Naturally plan: eating a healthy diet, getting plenty of physical activity, not smoking, maintaining a healthy body weight, and keeping blood pressure, cholesterol, and blood sugar at healthy levels. [49]

Success Story: *Anita Hirsch*

AGE: 75

HEIGHT: 5'6"

BLOOD PRESSURE IMPROVEMENT: Anita's systolic pressure dropped 29 points, and her diastolic pressure fell 9 points.

POUNDS LOST: 10½

"When I was younger, it didn't matter what I ate. I weighed 120 to 130 pounds, and it stayed like that," says Anita, a registered dietitian and recipe developer. "But my weight has been slowly going up, and I've noticed more fat in my stomach area, the place that's bad for your heart. It worried me."

Anita was motivated to take action when her doctor prescribed medication for her blood pressure in the winter of 2012. "I didn't want to take medication, but nothing else was helping," she notes. "The medicine did bring it down—and also reduced the number of migraine headaches I get—but I worry about side effects. I don't want to have to take more drugs and higher doses."

Dropping more than 10 pounds in 6 weeks and losing inches from her waist and hips feels great—and it shows, she says. "People have been saying, 'I think you've lost weight.' They see it in my face. When I stand and look at myself in the mirror, I am thinner." Enough so that it was time for a shopping trip for new clothes. "My daughter, who's my fashionista, picked out a pair of pants for me, and I don't even need a shaper underneath."

Health conscious at home and in her work, she's thrilled with her lower blood pressure numbers. At the start of the plan, Anita's blood pressure was 145/80 (high enough to be considered hypertensive) even with medication. After 4 weeks, it fell to a healthy 119/68. At the end of the 6-week plan, her final, official BP reading was 116/71, an optimal level that significantly reduces her risk for a heart attack or stroke. A 10-point drop in systolic blood pressure (the top number) or a 5-point drop in diastolic pressure (the bottom number) lowers heart attack risk 22 percent and stroke risk by a whopping 41 percent.[50] Since Anita's numbers dropped more than twice as far, she's slashed her risk even more.

Strength training and regular walking made her feel stronger and slimmer. "I spend a lot of time at the New Jersey shore in the summer," she says. "I would walk from our house to the water and back—a longer walk than you might think because there's about a mile of beach before you get to the ocean. I felt good. And running up and down the steps getting things ready for guests felt easier, too."

Her favorite foods on the plan? "I liked the Fiesta Shrimp Tacos (page 114), the Corn Tortilla Pizzas (page 120), and the Veggie and Cheddar Frittata (page 113). My son loved the Garlic-Ginger Tofu Stir-Fry (page 116). And the Peaches and Cream Hot Quinoa Cereal (page 87) was my favorite breakfast. I thought everything tasted good!" That includes the Green Machine Smoothie (page 88). "I've tested plenty of green drinks in my work as a recipe tester, but in the past I've just taken a few sips," she says. "Finally, I drank the whole thing. It was tasty and filling."

The plan's flexibility came in handy when Anita's husband was hospitalized for a week. "I was spending a lot of time visiting him," she says. "So I used a lot of the convenience food options with a salad or greens on the side. The frozen meals were a big help. I kept losing weight and my blood pressure kept going down."

CHAPTER 17

Track Your Success

Keeping track of your food choices, workouts, meditation practice, and blood pressure can make a difference for your weight and BP. Research shows that logging meals and movement can double weight loss.[1] Monitoring your blood pressure at home and keeping track of the numbers can nudge your pressure down a few extra points, too.

This is the place to do it. Keeping records with the simple forms in this chapter will help you stay motivated and accountable. You'll feel encouraged to keep on making great choices, notice backsliding more quickly, and see inspiring progress.

To keep track, just fill in the blanks. Don't forget to check your blood pressure once or twice a day (or more often if recommended by your doctor) and record the numbers. There is also a space for you to note your stress and energy levels. Once a week, weigh yourself and take basic measurements (chest, waist, hips) with a tape measure. We've included a week's worth of journal pages for Phase 1 and a sample page for Phase 2 that you can copy.

Taking Your Blood Pressure at Home
Studies show that the way you check your blood pressure can significantly affect the reading. These tips will help.

- Take your readings at the same time of day.
- Don't drink coffee (or caffeinated tea or soda), don't have tobacco, and don't exercise for at least 30 minutes before taking a reading.

- Empty your bladder beforehand (a full bladder raises BP).
- Sit in a chair with your back supported and your feet flat on the floor. Don't cross your legs. Relax for 5 minutes before taking your blood pressure.
- Keep your arm at heart level, relaxed, and supported on a table or on the armrest of a chair.
- Measure with short sleeves or a sleeveless shirt.
- If your BP is unusually elevated, wait 1 to 2 hours and repeat the measurement.

What to write down: A BP reading is two numbers.

1. **Systolic blood pressure.** This is the top or first number in your reading. It measures pressure on your arteries during a heartbeat. It's the higher of the two numbers.
2. **Diastolic blood pressure.** This is the bottom or second number in your reading. It measures pressure when your heart rests between beats. It's the lower of the two numbers.

Always record the systolic reading as the first number and the diastolic reading as the second number. For example, if your monitor shows that your blood pressure reading is 118/78, you would write **118/78** in your log.

Phase 1 Journal: Day 1

Date: _____

Beginning weight: _____

BEGINNING MEASUREMENTS

Chest: _____

Hips: _____

Waist: _____

MEALS

1. _____

_____

2. _____

_____

3. _____

_____

4. _____

_____

Other food: _____

_____

EXERCISE

Today I did:

____Interval Walk ____Steady-Paced Walk

I chose this Blood Pressure Bonus:

___Strength Training

___Energizing Yoga Routine

___Restorative Yoga Routine

I did the 5-Minute Meditation ____Yes ____No

Stress Level: ____High ____Medium ____Low

Energy Level: ____High ____Medium ____Low

BLOOD PRESSURE

Today I checked my blood pressure ____Yes ____No

MY READINGS (HOW MANY I DID TODAY)

DATE	TIME	BLOOD PRESSURE SYSTOLIC/DIASTOLIC	COMMENTS

Phase 1 Journal: Day 2

Date: _____

MEALS

1. _____

_____

2. _____

_____

3. _____

_____

4. _____

_____

Other food: _____

_____

EXERCISE

Today I did:

_____Interval Walk _____Steady-Paced Walk

I chose this Blood Pressure Bonus:

_____Strength Training

_____Energizing Yoga Routine

_____Restorative Yoga Routine

I did the 5-Minute Meditation ____Yes ____No

Stress Level: ___High ___Medium ___Low

Energy Level: ___High ___Medium ___Low

BLOOD PRESSURE

Today I checked my blood pressure ___Yes ___No

MY READINGS (HOW MANY I DID TODAY)

DATE	TIME	BLOOD PRESSURE SYSTOLIC/DIASTOLIC	COMMENTS

Phase 1 Journal: Day 3

Date: _____

MEALS

1. _____

_____

2. _____

_____

3. _____

_____

4. _____

_____

Other food: _____

_____

EXERCISE

Today I did:

_____Interval Walk _____Steady-Paced Walk

I chose this Blood Pressure Bonus:

_____Strength Training

_____Energizing Yoga Routine

_____Restorative Yoga Routine

I did the 5-Minute Meditation ____Yes ____No

Stress Level: ___High ___Medium ___Low

Energy Level: ___High ___Medium ___Low

BLOOD PRESSURE

Today I checked my blood pressure ___Yes ___No

MY READINGS (HOW MANY I DID TODAY)

DATE	TIME	BLOOD PRESSURE SYSTOLIC/DIASTOLIC	COMMENTS

Phase 1 Journal: Day 4

Date: _____

MEALS

1. _____

_____

2. _____

_____

3. _____

_____

4. _____

_____

Other food: _____

_____

EXERCISE

Today I did:

_____Interval Walk _____Steady-Paced Walk

I chose this Blood Pressure Bonus:

_____Strength Training

_____Energizing Yoga Routine

_____Restorative Yoga Routine

I did the 5-Minute Meditation _____Yes _____No

Stress Level: ___High ___Medium ___Low

Energy Level: ___High ___Medium ___Low

BLOOD PRESSURE

Today I checked my blood pressure ___Yes ___No

MY READINGS (HOW MANY I DID TODAY)

DATE	TIME	BLOOD PRESSURE SYSTOLIC/DIASTOLIC	COMMENTS

Phase 1 Journal: Day 5

Date: _____

MEALS

1. _____

_____

2. _____

_____

3. _____

_____

4. _____

_____

Other food: _____

_____

EXERCISE

Today I did:

_____Interval Walk _____Steady-Paced Walk

I chose this Blood Pressure Bonus:

_____Strength Training

_____Energizing Yoga Routine

_____Restorative Yoga Routine

I did the 5-Minute Meditation ____Yes ____No

Stress Level: ___High ___Medium ___Low

Energy Level: ___High ___Medium ___Low

BLOOD PRESSURE

Today I checked my blood pressure ___Yes ___No

MY READINGS (HOW MANY I DID TODAY)

DATE	TIME	BLOOD PRESSURE SYSTOLIC/DIASTOLIC	COMMENTS

Phase 1 Journal: Day 6

Date: _____

MEALS

1. _____

_____

2. _____

_____

3. _____

_____

4. _____

_____

Other food: _____

_____

EXERCISE

Today I did:

_____Interval Walk _____Steady-Paced Walk

I chose this Blood Pressure Bonus:

_____Strength Training

_____Energizing Yoga Routine

_____Restorative Yoga Routine

I did the 5-Minute Meditation ____Yes ____No

Stress Level: ___High ___Medium ___Low

Energy Level: ___High ___Medium ___Low

BLOOD PRESSURE

Today I checked my blood pressure ___Yes ___No

MY READINGS (HOW MANY I DID TODAY)

DATE	TIME	BLOOD PRESSURE SYSTOLIC/DIASTOLIC	COMMENTS

Phase 1 Journal: Day 7

Date: _____

MEALS

1. _____

_____

2. _____

_____

3. _____

_____

4. _____

_____

Other food: _____

_____

EXERCISE

Today I did:

_____Interval Walk _____Steady-Paced Walk

I chose this Blood Pressure Bonus:

_____Strength Training

_____Energizing Yoga Routine

_____Restorative Yoga Routine

I did the 5-Minute Meditation _____Yes _____No

Stress Level: ___High ___Medium ___Low

Energy Level: ___High ___Medium ___Low

BLOOD PRESSURE

Today I checked my blood pressure ___Yes ___No

MY READINGS (HOW MANY I DID TODAY)

DATE	TIME	BLOOD PRESSURE SYSTOLIC/DIASTOLIC	COMMENTS

Phase 2 Journal: Day _____

Date: _____

Beginning weight: _____

MEASUREMENTS AT THE START OF THE WEEK

Chest: _____

Hips: _____

Waist: _____

MEALS

1. My Phase 1 meal: _____

_____

My other three meal choices:

2. _____

_____

3. _____

_____

4. _____

_____

I had this Power Mineral Smoothie or Power Mineral Dessert: _____

_____

EXERCISE

Today I did:

_____Interval Walk _____Steady-Paced Walk

I chose this Blood Pressure Bonus:

___Strength Training

___Energizing Yoga Routine

___Restorative Yoga Routine

I did the 5-Minute Meditation ____Yes ____No

Stress Level: ____High ____Medium ____Low

Energy Level: ____High ____Medium ____Low

BLOOD PRESSURE

Today I checked my blood pressure ____Yes ____No

MY READINGS (HOW MANY I DID TODAY)

(We recommend checking one or two times a day. Check more often if recommended by your doctor.)

DATE	TIME	BLOOD PRESSURE SYSTOLIC/DIASTOLIC	COMMENTS

CHAPTER 18

Beyond Week 6: Maintaining the New You

It's time to celebrate! You've successfully completed the Lower Your Blood Pressure Naturally plan. You've lost weight, trimmed inches, and lowered your blood pressure. Plus, you feel more relaxed and energized than you have in years. What now?

Keep it up, of course.

You already know how. The last 6 weeks have taught you the skills and have introduced you to the foods that will allow you to maintain your new weight, size, and blood pressure level and that will help protect you from heart disease and stroke. Here's how to keep the healthy, sexy synergy of the plan's eight strategies going in your life.

Keep Your Sodium Intake Down and Your Power Mineral Intake High

Stock your kitchen with low-sodium Power Foods rich in calcium, magnesium, and potassium—the minerals that support healthier blood pressure. Reach for them at breakfast, lunch, and dinner and for snacks. Make them your go-to, grab-in-seconds first choice. Keep skim milk and yogurt in the fridge, stock your freezer with frozen peach slices, fill your fruit bowl with bananas. Prechop red bell peppers and broccoli for quick side dishes and for raw snacks. And reach for avocado instead of mayo for sandwiches and instead of processed dressings for salads. Top protein picks? Keep no-salt-added white beans in your cabinet, and stock your freezer with pork tenderloin and frozen tilapia fillets for quick dinners.

In a big hurry? Eat smart to avoid the biggest source of sodium in the American diet: convenience foods (like processed and packaged supermarket entrées and side dishes as well as fast food and restaurant fare). With a little planning, you can sidestep sodium, even when you don't have time to cook from scratch. Follow the tips in Chapter 10 to find lower-sodium options at restaurants and fast-food chains and to pair lower-sodium convenience foods with mineral-rich sides for superquick, nutritious dinners.

And keep using our low- and no-sodium spice blends in Chapter 8 to add flavor to the foods you prepare at home.

Choose These Mineral-Packed Foods, Too

In addition to our Power Foods—each one of which is rich in two out of three Power Minerals—know how to spot other mineral-packed, BP-friendly foods at the supermarket, at parties and picnics, and in restaurants. Eat plenty of these daily.

Potassium All-Stars

You need 4,700 milligrams of potassium a day for good health and good blood pressure control. Like the potassium-rich Power Foods, these foods deliver plenty of potassium.

FOOD	SERVING SIZE	POTASSIUM (MG)
Swiss chard	1 cup cooked	960
Lima beans	1 cup cooked	955
Potatoes	1 baked	925
Soybeans	1 cup cooked	885
Spinach	1 cup cooked	838
Lentils	1 cup cooked	730

(continued)

FOOD	SERVING SIZE	POTASSIUM (MG)
Kidney beans	1 cup cooked	716
Dried peas	1 cup cooked	709
Cod	4 ounces	586
Scallops	4 ounces	539
Winter squash	1 cup baked	494
Beets	1 cup cooked	442
Cantaloupe	1 cup	427
Tomatoes	1 cup raw	426
Carrots	1 cup raw	390
Green peas	1 cup raw	373
Fennel	1 cup raw	360
Brussels sprouts	1 cup raw	342
Blackstrap molasses	2 teaspoons	340
Cauliflower	1 cup raw	319

Calcium All-Stars

Keep enjoying calcium-rich Power Foods—skim milk and yogurt as well as white beans, kale, and broccoli. But don't stop there. Add these calcium all-stars to your plate regularly. You need 1,200 milligrams of this mineral daily.

FOOD	SERVING SIZE	CALCIUM (MG)
Sardines	3 ounces	346
Collard greens	1 cup cooked	266
Tofu	½ cup	258
Turnip greens	1 cup cooked	197
Rhubarb	½ cup cooked	174

FOOD	SERVING SIZE	CALCIUM (MG)
Scallops	4 ounces	130
Blackstrap molasses	2 teaspoons	117
Spinach	½ cup cooked	115
Mustard greens	1 cup cooked	103
Swiss chard	1 cup cooked	101
Bok choy	½ cup cooked	79
Pinto beans	½ cup cooked	45
Red beans	½ cup cooked	41

Magnesium All-Stars

Aim for 420 milligrams of this Power Mineral daily. In addition to magnesium-rich Power Foods—like avocado, yogurt, and bananas—reach for these regularly.

FOOD	SERVING SIZE	MAGNESIUM (MG)
Almonds, dry roasted	1 ounce	80
Spinach	½ cup cooked	78
Cashews, dry roasted	1 ounce	74
Shredded wheat cereal	2 large biscuits	61
Soy milk, plain or vanilla	1 cup	61
Black beans	½ cup cooked	60
Soybeans	½ cup cooked	50
Peanut butter	2 tablespoons	49
Whole wheat bread	2 slices	46
Potato, baked with skin	1 medium	43
Brown rice	½ cup cooked	42

(continued)

FOOD	SERVING SIZE	MAGNESIUM (MG)
Kidney beans	½ cup cooked	35
Salmon	3 ounces	26
Halibut	3 ounces	24
Chicken breast	3 ounces	22
Apple	1 medium	9
Carrot	1 medium	7

Take a Walk

Got 10 minutes? That's all you need to start reaping the blood pressure benefits of walking. As you discovered in this plan, taking three 10-minute walks a day (or two 15-minute walks) helps your BP as much or more than taking one continuous 30-minute walk. Never cheat yourself out of all the perks that walking provides. Work in a 20-minute interval walk three times a week, as well, if your doctor has okayed it. The bursts of faster-paced movement help you burn more fat and calories and help your heart even more than steady-paced walking.

Treat Yourself to a Daily Blood Pressure Bonus

You deserve it! Keep up with strength training and yoga. In just 15 minutes a day, you'll continue building strong, toned muscle and busting stress. These blood pressure essentials also help burn calories and, by easing tension, can help you avoid emotional eating that leads to weight regain. Fit in a daily 5-minute meditation, too.

Track Your Meals, Exercise, and Blood Pressure

Logging isn't just for dieters. Continuing to keep track of your meals, your workouts, and your daily blood pressure numbers will motivate you to keep making great choices. You'll stay slimmer and stronger, and you'll lower your risk for blood pressure problems that raise risk for heart attacks and strokes.

Endnotes

Chapter 1

1 National Institute of Neurological Disorders and Stroke, "Brain Basics: Preventing Stroke," NIH Publication No. 11-3440b, www.ninds.nih.gov/disorders/stroke/preventing_stroke.htm.

2 A. Go et al., "Heart Disease and Stroke Statistics—2013 Update: A Report from the American Heart Association," *Circulation* 127, no. 1 (January 1, 2013): e6–e245.

3 R. Khanna et al., "Missed Opportunities for Treatment of Uncontrolled Hypertension at Physician Office Visits in the United States, 2005 through 2009, *Archives of Internal Medicine* 172, no. 17 (2012): 1344–45.

4 Centers for Disease Control and Prevention, "FastStats: Ambulatory Care Use and Physician Visits," www.cdc.gov/nchs/fastats/docvisit.htm.

5 Centers for Disease Control and Prevention, "FastStats: Hypertension," www.cdc.gov/nchs/fastats/hyprtens.htm.

6 P. Yoon et al., "Control of Hypertension among Adults—National Health and Nutrition Examination Survey, United States, 2005-2008," supplement, *Morbidity and Mortality Weekly Report (MMWR)* 62, no. S2 (June 15, 2012): S19–S25.

7 B. Egan et al., "Blood Pressure and Cholesterol Control in Hypertensive Hypercholesterolemic Patients," *Circulation* 128 (2013): 29–41.

8 Centers for Disease Control and Prevention, "CDC Vital Signs: High Blood Pressure Is Out of Control for Too Many Americans," press briefing transcript, September 4, 2012, www.cdc.gov/media/releases /2012/t0904_hypertension.html.

9 Yoon et al., "Control of Hypertension among Adults."

Chapter 2

1 Centers for Disease Control and Prevention, "High Blood Pressure Fact Sheet," www.cdc.gov/dhdsp/data1/4statistics/fact1/4sheets/fs1/4bloodpressure.htm.

2 E. P. Jolles et al., "A Qualitative Study of Patient Perspectives about Hypertension," *ISRN Hypertension* 2013 (2013): 1–10.

3 B. Williams, L. H. Lindholm, and P. Sever, "Systolic Pressure Is All That Matters," *Lancet* 371, no. 9631 (June 28, 2008): 2219–21.

4 W. White, "Importance of Blood Pressure Control Over a 24-Hour Period," supplement, *Journal of Managed Care Pharmacy* 13, no. 8, S-b (October 2007): S34–S39.

5 Ibid.

6 L. García-Ortiz et al., "Blood Pressure Circadian Pattern and Physical Exercise Assessment by Accelerometer and 7-Day Physical Activity Recall Scale," *American Journal of Hypertension* (August 24, 2013), http://ajh.oxfordjournals.org/content/early/2013/08/24/ajh.hpt159.abstract.

7 J. M. Neutel et al., "Magnitude of the Early Morning Blood Pressure Surge in Untreated Hypertensive Patients: A Pooled Analysis," *International Journal of Clinical Practice* 62, no. 11 (November 2008): 1654–63.

8 M. Y. Rhee et al., "Elevation of Morning Blood Pressure in Sodium Resistant Subjects by High Sodium Diet," *Journal of Korean Medical Science* 28, no. 4 (April 2013): 555–63.

9 T. J. Moore et al., "Effect of Dietary Patterns on Ambulatory Blood Pressure: Results from the Dietary Approaches to Stop Hypertension (DASH) Trial," *Hypertension* 34 (1999): 472–77.

10 A. Agarwal, G. H. Williams, and N. D. Fisher, "Genetics of Human Hypertension," *Trends in Endocrinology and Metabolism* 16, no. 3 (April 2005): 127–33.

11 New York-Presbyterian Hospital, "Why African Americans Are at Greater Risk of Hypertension and Kidney Disease," July 13, 2009, http://nyp.org/news/hospital/risk-hypertension-kidney-disease.html.

12 G. Howard et al., "Racial Differences in the Impact of Elevated Systolic Blood Pressure on Stroke Risk," *JAMA Internal Medicine* 173, no. 1 (January 14, 2013): 46–51.

13 F. D. Fuchs, "Why Do Black Americans Have Higher Prevalence of Hypertension? An Enigma Still Unsolved," *Hypertension* 57 (2011): 379–80.

14 P. K. Whelton et al., "Sodium Reduction and Weight Loss in the Treatment of Hypertension in Older Persons: A Randomized Controlled Trial of Nonpharmacologic Interventions in the Elderly (TONE): TONE Collaborative Research Group," *JAMA* 279, no. 11 (March 18, 1998): 839–46.

15 W. J. Kostis et al., "Relationships between Selected Gene Polymorphisms and Blood Pressure Sensitivity to Weight Loss in Elderly Persons with Hypertension," *Hypertension* 61 (2013): 857–63.

16 National Institutes of Health, "NHLBI Study Finds DASH Diet and Reduced Sodium Lowers Blood Pressure for All," news release, December 17, 2001, www.nih.gov/news/pr/dec2001/nhlbi-17.htm.

17 R. S. Vasan et al., "Residual Lifetime Risk for Developing Hypertension in Middle-Aged Women and Men: The Framingham Heart Study," *JAMA* 287, no. 8 (February 27, 2002): 1003–10.

18 J. P. Forman et al., "Association between Sodium Intake and Change in Uric Acid, Urine Albumin Excretion, and the Risk of Developing Hypertension," *Circulation* 125 (2012): 3108–16.

19 A. Nunes Faria et al., "Impact of Visceral Fat on Blood Pressure and Insulin Sensitivity in Hypertensive Obese Women," *Obesity* 10, no. 12 (December 2002): 1203–6.

20 L. Svetkey, "Hypertension Grand Rounds," *Hypertension* 45 (2005): 1056–61.

21 H. D. Sesso et al., "Alcohol Consumption and the Risk of Hypertension in Women and Men," *Hypertension* 51, no. 4 (April 2008): 1080–87.

22 N. Kaplan, "Smoking and Hypertension," UpToDate, www.uptodate.com/contents/smoking-and-hypertension.

23 R. Nakanishi et al., "Coronary Artery Disease Extent, Severity and Risk among Active Smokers, Past Smokers and Non-Smokers: A Prospective Study of 13,372 Patients Undergoing Coronary CT Angiography," abstract, supplement, *European Heart Journal* 34, no. S1 (2013), doi: 10.1093/eurheartj/eht308.P2071.

24 A. Go et al., "Heart Disease and Stroke Statistics—2013 Update: A Report from the American Heart Association," *Circulation* 127, no. 1 (January 1, 2013): e6–e245.

25 M. Madhur et al., "Hypertension: Prognosis," Medscape, http://emedicine.medscape.com /article/241381-overview#aw2aab6b2b6aa.

26 S. L. Bacon et al., "The Role of Ischaemia and Pain in the Blood Pressure Response to Exercise Stress Testing in Patients with Coronary Heart Disease," *Journal of Human Hypertension* 20, no. 9 (2006): 672–78.

27 Go et al., "Heart Disease and Stroke Statistics—2013 Update."

28 D. Brown, W. Giles, and K. Greenlund, "Blood Pressure Parameters and Risk of Fatal Stroke, NHANES II Mortality Study," *American Journal of Hypertension* 20, no. 3 (March 2007): 338–41.

29 M. Lee et al., "Presence of Baseline Prehypertension and Risk of Incident Stroke: A Meta-Analysis," *Neurology* 77 (2011): 1330–37.

30 J. Segura et al., "High Prevalence of Target Organ Damage in Hypertensive and Prehypertensive Patients with Associated Cardiovascular Risk Factors," *Journal of Hypertension* 28 (June 2010): e466.

31 Johns Hopkins Medicine Health Alerts, "How Hypertension Can Put Your Vision at Risk," July 29, 2011, www.johnshopkinshealthalerts.com/alerts/vision/hypertension-vision-connection1/45796-1.html.

32 S. Debette et al., "Midlife Vascular Risk Factor Exposure Accelerates Structural Brain Aging and Cognitive Decline," *Neurology* 77, no. 5 (August 2, 2011): 461–68.

33 D. S. Silverberg, A. Iaina, and A. Oksenberg, "Treating Obstructive Sleep Apnea Improves Essential Hypertension and Quality of Life," *American Family Physician* 65, no. 2 (January 15, 2002): 229–37.

34 A. Roth et al., "Prevalence and Risk Factors for Erectile Dysfunction in Men with Diabetes, Hypertension, or Both Diseases: A Community Survey among 1,412 Israeli Men," *Clinical Cardiology* 26, no. 1 (January 2003): 25–30.

35 R. Caudarella et al., "Salt Intake, Hypertension, and Osteoporosis," supplement, *Journal of Endocrinological Investigation* 32, no. S4 (2009): S15–S20.

36 M. Varenna et al., "The Association between Osteoporosis and Hypertension: The Role of a Low Dairy Intake," *Calcified Tissue International* 93, no. 1 (July 2013): 86–92.

Chapter 3

1 J. P. Forman et al., "Association between Sodium Intake and Change in Uric Acid, Urine Albumin Excretion, and the Risk of Developing Hypertension," *Circulation* 125 (2012): 3108–16.

2 A. Khosravi et al., "Salt Intake, Obesity, and Pre-hypertension among Iranian Adults: A Cross-Sectional Study," *Pakistan Journal of Medical Sciences* 28, no. 2 (January–March 2012): 297–302.

3 J. He Feng, J. Li, and G. MacGregor, "Effect of Longer Term Modest Salt Reduction on Blood Pressure: Cochrane Systematic Review and Meta-Analysis of Randomised Trials," *British Medical Journal* 346 (2013), doi: 10.1136/bmj.f1325.

4 Ibid.

5 University of Helsinki, "Salt Intake Is Strongly Associated with Obesity," *ScienceDaily*, November 13, 2006, www.sciencedaily.com/releases/2006/11/061101151027.htm.

6 A. Mozumdar and G. Liguori, "Persistent Increase of Prevalence of Metabolic Syndrome among U.S. Adults: NHANES III to NHANES 1999–2006," *Diabetes Care* 34, no. 1 (January 2011): 216–19.

7 E. Pimenta et al., "Effects of Dietary Sodium Reduction on Blood Pressure in Subjects with Resistant Hypertension: Results from a Randomized Trial," *Hypertension* 54, no. 3 (September 2009): 475–81.

8 Centers for Disease Control and Prevention (CDC), "*MMWR* Highlights," October 20, 2011, www.cdc.gov/Salt/pdfs/MMWR_Highlights_Sodium_Intake_2011.pdf.

9 M. K. Hoy et al., "Sodium Intake of the U.S. Population: What We Eat in America, NHANES 2007–2008," US Department of Agriculture, October 2011, www.ars.usda.gov/sp2userfiles/place /12355000/pdf/dbrief/sodium_intake_0708.pdf.

10 International Food Information Council Foundation, "IFIC Review: Sodium in Food and Health," Food Insight, April 20, 2010, www.foodinsight.org/Resources/Detail.aspx?topic=IFIC_Review_ Sodium_in_Food_and_Health.

11 E. S. Ford and A. H. Mokdad, "Dietary Magnesium Intake in a National Sample of U.S. Adults," *Journal of Nutrition* 133, no. 9 (September 1, 2003): 2879–82.

12 R. L. Bailey et al., "Estimation of Total Usual Calcium and Vitamin D Intakes in the United States," *Journal of Nutrition* 140, no 4 (April 2010): 817–22.

13 N. R. Cook et al., "Joint Effects of Sodium and Potassium Intake on Subsequent Cardiovascular Disease: The Trials of Hypertension Prevention Follow-up Study, *Archives of Internal Medicine* 169, no. 1 (January 12, 2009): 32–40.

14 W. J. Kostis et al., "Relationships between Selected Gene Polymorphisms and Blood Pressure Sensitivity to Weight Loss in Elderly Persons with Hypertension," *Hypertension* 61 (2013): 857–63.

15 G. Yang, "Salt Intake in Individuals with Metabolic Syndrome," *Lancet* 373, no. 9666 (March 2009): 792–94.

16 Medical College of Georgia, "Connection Elucidated between Obesity, Salt Sensitivity and High Blood Pressure," *ScienceDaily*, June 18, 2010, www.sciencedaily.com/releases/2010/06/100617102725.htm.

17 American Heart Association, "Physical Activity Decreases Salt's Effect on Blood Pressure," March 23, 2011, http://newsroom.heart.org/pr/aha/1289.aspx.

18 Critique based on P. K. Whelton, "Urinary Sodium and Cardiovascular Disease Risk: Informing Guidelines for Sodium Consumption," *JAMA* 306, no. 20 (November 2011): 2262–64; and R. S. Taylor et al., "Reduced Dietary Salt for the Prevention of Cardiovascular Disease: A Meta-Analysis of Randomized Controlled Trials (Cochrane Review)," *American Journal of Hypertension* 24, no. 8 (August 2011): 843–53.

19 Ibid.

20 N. A. Graudal, T. Hubeck-Graudal, and G. Jurgens, "Effects of Low Sodium Diet versus High Sodium Diet on Blood Pressure, Renin, Aldosterone, Catecholamines, Cholesterol, and Triglyceride (Cochrane Review)," *American Journal of Hypertension* 25, no. 1 (2012): 1–15.

21 M. J. O'Donnell et al., "Urinary Sodium and Potassium Excretion and Risk of Cardiovascular Events," *JAMA* 306, no. 20 (November 2011): 2229–38.

22 Harvey V. Fineberg letter to Kathleen Sibelius, http://cspinet.org/new/pdf/iom_fineberg_letter _to_sibelius06032013.pdf.

23 Center for Science in the Public Interest, "Institute of Medicine Chief Knocks Press Coverage of Salt Report," June 17, 2013, www.cspinet.org/new/201306171.html.

24 M. F. Jacobson, "The *New York Times* Bungles the Latest Salt Report," *The Blog, Huffington Post*, May 20, 2013, www.huffingtonpost.com/michael-f-jacobson/sodium-health_b_3294901.html.

25 F. D. Fuchs et al., "Prevention of Hypertension in Patients with Prehypertension: Protocol for the PREVER-Prevention Trial," *Trials* 12, no. 65 (2011): 1–7.

26 P. M. Kris-Etherton et al., "Milk Products, Dietary Patterns and Blood Pressure Management," *Journal of the American College of Nutrition*, supplement, 28, no. S1 (February 2009): S103–S119.

27 Forman et al., "Association between Sodium Intake and Change in Uric Acid."

28 CDC, "*MMWR* Highlights."

29 S. Burton et al., "Attacking the Obesity Epidemic: The Potential Health Benefits of Providing Nutrition Information in Restaurants," *American Journal of Public Health* 96, no. 9 (September 2006): 1669–75.

30 A. J. Moshfegh et al., "Vital Signs: Food Categories Contributing the Most to Sodium Consumption—United States, 2007–2008," *Morbidity and Mortality Weekly Report* 61, no. 5 (2012): 92–98.

31 M. F. Jacobson, S. Havas, and R. McCarter, "Changes in Sodium Levels in Processed and Restaurant Foods, 2005 to 2011," *JAMA Internal Medicine* 173, no. 14 (July 22, 2013): 1285–91.

32 M. J. Scourboutakos, Z. Semnani-Azad, and M. R. L'Abbe, "Restaurant Meals: Almost a Full Day's Worth of Calories, Fats, and Sodium," *JAMA Internal Medicine* 173, no. 14 (July 2013): 1373–74.

33 J. Arcand et al., "Evaluation of Sodium Levels in Hospital Patient Menus," *Archives of Internal Medicine* 172, no. 16 (September 10, 2012): 1261–62.

34 M. Bertino, G. K. Beauchamp, and K. Engelman, "Long-Term Reduction in Dietary Sodium Alters the Taste of Salt," *American Journal of Clinical Nutrition* 36, no. 6 (December 1982): 1134–44.

Chapter 4

1 A. Drewnowski, M. Maillot, and C. Rehm, "Reducing the Sodium-Potassium Ratio in the US Diet: A Challenge for Public Health," *American Journal of Clinical Nutrition* 96, no. 2 (August 2012): 439–44.

2 M. K. Hoy and J. D. Goldman, "Potassium Intake of the U.S. Population: What We Eat in America, NHANES 2009–2010," US Department of Agriculture, September 2010, www.ars.usda.gov /SP2UserFiles/Place/12355000/pdf/DBrief/10_potassium_intake_0910.pdf.

3 N. R. Cook et al., "Joint Effects of Sodium and Potassium Intake on Subsequent Cardiovascular Disease: The Trials of Hypertension Prevention (TOHP) Follow-up Study," *Archives of Internal Medicine* 169, no. 1 (January 12, 2009): 32–40.

4 Q. Yang et al., "Sodium and Potassium Intake and Mortality Among US Adults," *Archives of Internal Medicine* 171, no. 13 (July 11, 2011): 1183–91.

5 F. J. Haddy, P. M. Vanhoutte, and M. Feletou, "Role of Potassium in Regulating Blood Flow and Blood Pressure," *American Journal of Physiology Regulatory, Integrative and Comparative Physiology* 290, no. 3 (March 2006): R546–R52.

6 Ibid.

7 Yang et al., "Sodium and Potassium Intake and Mortality."

8 National Institutes of Health Office of Dietary Supplements, "Calcium," http://ods.od.nih.gov /factsheets/Calcium-HealthProfessional/.

9 P. M. Kris-Etherton et al., "Milk Products, Dietary Patterns and Blood Pressure Management," supplement, *Journal of the American College of Nutrition* 28, no. S1 (February 2009): S103–S119.

10 I. M. Hajjar et al., "Dietary Calcium Lowers the Age-Related Rise in Blood Pressure in the United States: The NHANES III Survey," *Journal of Clinical Hypertension* 5, no. 2 (March–April 2003): 122–26.

11 M. Van Hemelrijck et al., "Calcium Intake and Serum Concentration in Relation to Risk of Cardiovascular Death in NHANES III," *PLOS ONE* 8, no. 4 (April 2013), www.plosone.org/article /info%3Adoi%2F10.1371%2Fjournal.pone.0061037.

12 Q. Xiao et al., "Dietary and Supplemental Calcium Intake and Cardiovascular Disease Mortality:

The National Institutes of Health-AARP Diet and Health Study," *JAMA Internal Medicine* 173, no. 8 (April 22, 2013): 639–46.

13 K. Pentti et al., "Use of Calcium Supplements and the Risk of Coronary Heart Disease in 52-62-Year-Old Women: The Kuopio Osteoporosis Risk Factor and Prevention Study," *Maturitas* 63, no. 1 (May 20, 2009): 73–78.

14 Van Hemelrijck et al., "Calcium Intake and Serum Concentration."

15 K. Michaëlsson et al., "Long Term Calcium Intake and Rates of All Cause and Cardiovascular Mortality: Community Based Prospective Longitudinal Cohort Study," *British Medical Journal* 346 (February 13, 2013), doi: 10.1136/bmj.f228.

16 Institute of Medicine, "Dietary Reference Intakes for Calcium and Vitamin D," November 2010, www.iom.edu/~/media/Files/Report%20Files/2010/Dietary-Reference-Intakes-for-Calcium-and -Vitamin-D/Vitamin%20D%20and%20Calcium%202010%20Report%20Brief.pdf.

17 R. L. Bailey et al., "Estimation of Total Usual Calcium and Vitamin D Intakes in the United States," *Journal of Nutrition* 140, no. 4 (April 2010): 817–22.

18 Kris-Etherton et al., "Milk Products, Dietary Patterns and Blood Pressure Management."

19 J. B. Brill, "Lifestyle Intervention Strategies for the Prevention and Treatment of Hypertension: A Review," *American Journal of Lifestyle Medicine* 5, no. 4 (July–August 2011): 346–60.

20 Kris-Etherton et al., "Milk Products, Dietary Patterns and Blood Pressure Management."

21 Oregon State University, Linus Pauling Institute, Micronutrient Information Center, "Magnesium," http://lpi.oregonstate.edu/infocenter/minerals/magnesium/.

22 M. M. Joosten et al., "Urinary Magnesium Excretion and Risk of Hypertension: The Prevention of Renal and Vascular End-Stage Disease Study," *Hypertension* 61, no. 6 (June 2013): 1161–67.

23 Ibid.

24 Ibid.

25 A. Ascherio et al., "A Prospective Study of Nutritional Factors and Hypertension among US Men," *Circulation* 86, no. 5 (November 1992): 1475–84; and A. Ascherio et al., "Prospective Study of Nutritional Factors, Blood Pressure, and Hypertension among US Women," *Hypertension* 27, no. 5 (May 1996): 1065–72.

26 J. M. Peacock et al., "Relationship of Serum and Dietary Magnesium to Incident Hypertension: The Atherosclerosis Risk in Communities (ARIC) Study," *Annals of Epidemiology* 9, no. 3 (April 1999): 159–65.

27 E. S. Ford and A. H. Mokdad, "Dietary Magnesium Intake in a National Sample of U.S. Adults," *Journal of Nutrition* 133, no. 9 (September 1, 2003): 2879–82.

28 National Institutes of Health Office of Dietary Supplements, "Magnesium," http://ods.od.nih.gov /factsheets/Magnesium-HealthProfessional/.

29 Brill, "Lifestyle Intervention Strategies for the Prevention and Treatment of Hypertension."

Chapter 5

1 P. K. Whelton et al., "Sodium Reduction and Weight Loss in the Treatment of Hypertension in Older Persons: A Randomized Controlled Trial of Nonpharmacologic Interventions in the Elderly (TONE)," *JAMA* 279, no. 11 (March 18, 1998): 839–46.

2 Ibid.

3 International Food Information Council Foundation, "IFIC Review: Sodium in Food and Health,"

Food Insight, April 20, 2010, www.foodinsight.org/Resources/Detail.aspx?topic=IFIC1/4Review1 /4Sodium1/4in1/4Food1/4and1/4Health.

4 Writing Group of the PREMIER Collaborative Research Group, "Effects of Comprehensive Lifestyle Modification on Blood Pressure Control: Main Results of the PREMIER Clinical Trial," *JAMA* 289, no. 16 (April 2003): 2083–93.

5 T. A. Kotchen, "Obesity-Related Hypertension: Epidemiology, Pathophysiology, and Clinical Management," *American Journal of Hypertension* 23, no. 11 (November 2010): 1170–78.

6 D. W. Harsha and G. A. Bray, "Controversies in Hypertension: Weight Loss and Blood Pressure Control (Pro)," *Hypertension* 51 (2008): 1420–25.

7 Ibid.

8 T. A. Kotchen, "Obesity-Related Hypertension: Epidemiology, Pathophysiology, and Clinical Management," *American Journal of Hypertension* 23, no. 11 (November 2010): 1170–78.

9 D. A. Levine et al., "Moderate Waist Circumference and Hypertension Prevalence: The REGARDS Study," *American Journal of Hypertension* 24, no. 4 (April 2011): 482–88.

10 G. Yang et al., "Impacts of Weight Change on Prehypertension in Middle-Aged and Elderly Women," *International Journal of Obesity* 31, no. 12 (December 2007): 1818–25.

11 T. M. Frisoli et al., "Beyond Salt: Lifestyle Modifications and Blood Pressure," *European Heart Journal* 32, no. 24 (December 2011): 3081–87.

12 Harsha and Bray, "Controversies in Hypertension."

13 G. P. Shantha et al., "Intentional Weight Loss and Dose Reductions of Antihypertensive Medications: A Retrospective Cohort Study," *Cardiorenal Medicine* 3, no. 1 (April 2013): 17–25.

14 Frisoli et al., "Beyond Salt."

15 Kotchen, "Obesity-Related Hypertension."

16 Frisoli et al., "Beyond Salt."

17 Kotchen, "Obesity-Related Hypertension."

18 J. E. Neter et al., "Influence of Weight Reduction on Blood Pressure: A Meta-Analysis of Randomized Controlled Trials," *Hypertension* 42, no. 5 (November 2003): 878–84.

19 G. F. Fletcher et al., "Statement on Exercise: Benefits and Recommendations for Physical Activity Programs for All Americans," *Circulation* 94 (1996): 857–62.

20 E. G. Ciolac, "High-Intensity Interval Training and Hypertension: Maximizing the Benefits of Exercise?" *American Journal of Cardiovascular Disease* 2, no. 2 (2012): 102–10.

21 Ibid.

22 H. E. Molmen-Hansen et al., "Aerobic Interval Training Reduces Blood Pressure and Improves Myocardial Function in Hypertensive Patients," *European Journal of Preventive Cardiology* 19, no. 2 (April 2012): 151–60.

23 K. Nemoto et al., "Effects of High-Intensity Interval Walking Training on Physical Fitness and Blood Pressure in Middle-Aged and Older People," *Mayo Clinic Proceedings* 82, no. 7 (July 2007): 803–11, www.ncbi.nlm.nih.gov/pubmed/17605959.

24 A. E. Tjonna et al., "Aerobic Interval Training versus Continuous Moderate Exercise as a Treatment for the Metabolic Syndrome: A Pilot Study," *Circulation* 118, no. 4 (July 22, 2008): 346–54.

25 U. Wisloff, et al., "Exercise Physiology: Superior Cardiovascular Effect of Aerobic Interval Training versus Moderate Continuous Training in Heart Failure Patients, A Randomized Study," *Circulation* 115 (2007): 3086–94.

26 D. M. Bhammar, S. S. Angadi, and G. A. Gaesser, "Effects of Fractionized and Continuous Exercise on 24-h Ambulatory Blood Pressure," *Medicine and Science in Sports and Exercise* 44, no. 12 (December 2012): 2270–76.

27 T. Shiraev and G. Barclay, "Evidence Based Exercise: Clinical Benefits of High Intensity Interval Training," *AFP* 41, no. 12 (December 2012): 960–62.

28 J. Talanian et al., "Two Weeks of High-Intensity Aerobic Interval Training Increases the Capacity for Fat Oxidation during Exercise in Women," *Journal of Applied Physiology* 102, no. 4 (April 2007): 1439–47.

29 American College of Sports Medicine, "For All-Day Metabolism Boost, Try Interval Training," August 1, 2011, www.acsm.org/about-acsm/media-room/acsm-in-the-news/2011/08/01 /for-all-day-metabolism-boost-try-interval-training.

30 "High-Intensity Interval Training May Be Making a HIIT in Unsuspected Ways," *Fitnovatives* (blog), ACE, March 28, 2013, www.acefitness.org/blog/3207/.

31 Ciolac, "High-Intensity Interval Training and Hypertension."

32 W. L. Westcott et al., "Prescribing Physical Activity: Applying the ACSM Protocols for Exercise Type, Intensity, and Duration across 3 Training Frequencies," *Physician and Sportsmedicine* 37, no. 2 (June 2009): 51–58.

33 R. D. Brook et al., "Beyond Medications and Diet: Alternative Approaches to Lowering Blood Pressure: Scientific Statement from the American Heart Association," *Hypertension* 61 (2013): 1360–83.

34 M. R. Moraes et al., "Chronic Conventional Resistance Exercise Reduces Blood Pressure in Stage 1 Hypertensive Men," *Journal of Strength and Conditioning Research* 26, no. 4 (April 2012): 1122–29.

35 W. Westcott, "ACSM Strength Training Guidelines: Role in Body Composition and Health Enhancement," *ACSM's Health & Fitness Journal* 13, no. 4 (June 2009): 14–22.

36 W. L. Westcott and R. A. Winett, "Applying the ACSM Guidelines," *Fitness Management* 22, no. 1 (January 2006): 50–54.

37 D. L. Cohen et al., "Iyengar Yoga versus Enhanced Usual Care on Blood Pressure in Patients with Prehypertension to Stage I Hypertension: A Randomized Controlled Trial," *Evidence-Based Complementary and Alternative Medicine* 2011 (2011): 1–8.

38 C. Phend, "Yoga Can Bring Down BP a Bit," Medpage Today, May 27, 2013, www.medpagetoday.com /MeetingCoverage/ASH/39209.

39 Brook et al., "Beyond Medications and Diet."

40 K. Uhlig et al., "Self-Measured Blood Pressure Monitoring in the Management of Hypertension: A Systematic Review and Meta-Analysis," *Annals of Internal Medicine* 159, no. 3 (2013): 184–94.

Chapter 10

1 C. D. Chapman, "Lifestyle Determinants of the Drive to Eat: A Meta-Analysis," *American Journal of Clinical Nutrition* 92, no. 3 (September 2012): 492–97.

Chapter 11

1 A. V. Patel, "Leisure Time Spent Sitting in Relation to Total Mortality in a Prospective Cohort of US Adults," *American Journal of Epidemiology* 172, no. 4 (2010): 419–29.

2 Prevention.com Expert Center, "Featured Question: When Is the Best Time of the Day to Exercise?" www.prevention.com/best-time-exercise#ixzz22Qj8kwKD.

3 J. T. Manire et al., "Diurnal Variation of Hamstring and Lumbar Flexibility," *Journal of Strength and Conditioning Research* 24, no. 6 (June 2010): 1464–71.

4 American College of Sports Medicine, "Selecting and Effectively Using Hydration for Fitness," 2011, www.acsm.org/docs/brochures/selecting-and-effectively-using-hydration-for-fitness.pdf.

Chapter 15

1 J. W. Anderson, C. Liu, and R. J. Kryscio, "Blood Pressure Response to Transcendental Meditation: A Meta-Analysis," *American Journal of Hypertension* 21, no. 3 (March 2008): 310–16.

2 P. Palta et al., "Evaluation of a Mindfulness-Based Intervention Program to Decrease Blood Pressure in Low-Income African-American Older Adults," *Journal of Urban Health* 89, no. 2 (April 2012): 308–16.

3 S. Rosenzweig et al., "Mindfulness-Based Stress Reduction Is Associated with Improved Glycemic Control in Type 2 Diabetes Mellitus: A Pilot Study," *Alternative Therapies in Health and Medicine* 13, no. 5 (September–October 2007): 36–38.

4 T. S. Campbell et al., "Impact of Mindfulness-Based Stress Reduction (MBSR) on Attention, Rumination and Resting Blood Pressure in Women with Cancer: A Waitlist-Controlled Study," *Journal of Behavioral Medicine* 35, no. 3 (June 2012): 262–71.

5 L. E. Carlson et al., "One Year Pre-Post Intervention Follow-up of Psychological, Immune, Endocrine and Blood Pressure Outcomes of Mindfulness-Based Stress Reduction (MBSR) in Breast and Prostate Cancer Outpatients," *Brain, Behavior, and Immunity* 21, no. 8 (November 2007): 1038–49.

6 R. D. Brook et al., "Beyond Medications and Diet: Alternative Approaches to Lowering Blood Pressure; A Scientific Statement from the American Heart Association," *Hypertension* 61 (2013): 1360–83.

7 V. A. Barnes and D. W. Orme-Johnson, "Prevention and Treatment of Cardiovascular Disease in Adolescents and Adults through the Transcendental Meditation Program: A Research Review Update," *Current Hypertension Reviews* 8, no. 3 (August 2012): 227–42.

8 D. R. Young, et al., "The Effects of Aerobic Exercise and T'ai Chi on Blood Pressure in Older People: Results of a Randomized Trial," *Journal of the American Geriatric Society* 47, no. 3 (March 1999): 277–84.

9 G. Y. Yeh et al., "The Effect of Tai Chi Exercise on Blood Pressure: A Systematic Review," *Preventive Cardiology* 11, no. 2 (Spring 2008): 82–89.

10 J. Greenhalgh, R. Dickson, and Y. Dundar, "Biofeedback for Hypertension: A Systematic Review," *Journal of Hypertension* 28, no. 4 (April 2010): 644–52.

11 Resperate's Web site, www.resperate.com.

12 K. R. Mahtani, D. Nunan, and C. J. Heneghan, "Device-Guided Breathing Exercises in the Control of Human Blood Pressure: Systematic Review and Meta-Analysis," *Journal of Hypertension* 30, no. 5 (May 2012): 852–60.

13 E. A. Macklin et al., "Stop Hypertension with the Acupuncture Research Program (SHARP): Results of a Randomized, Controlled Clinical Trial," *Hypertension* 48, no. 5 (November 2006): 838–45.

14 Brook et al., "Beyond Medications and Diet."

15 M. Givi, "Durability of Effect of Massage Therapy on Blood Pressure," *International Journal of Preventive Medicine* 4, no. 5 (May 2013): 511–16.

16 M. S. Chaya et al., "The Effects of Hearty Extended Unconditional (HEU) Laughter Using Laughter Yoga Techniques on Physiological, Psychological, and Immunological Parameters in the Workplace: A Randomized Control Trial," reported at the American Society of Hypertension 2008 Annual Meeting, May 14, 2008, www.medpagetoday.com/MeetingCoverage/ASH/9484.

17 M. Salamon, "Laughter, Music May Lower Blood Pressure, Study Says," *US News & World Report: Health*, March 25, 2011, http://health.usnews.com/health-news/family-health/heart/articles/2011 /03/25/laughter-music-may-lower-blood-pressure-study-says.

18 S. A. Tan et al., "Humor, as an Adjunct Therapy in Cardiac Rehabilitation, Attenuates Catecholamines and Myocardial Infarction Recurrence," *Advances in Mind-Body Medicine* 22, no. 3–4 (Winter 2007): 8–12.

19 Salamon, "Laughter, Music May Lower Blood Pressure."

20 K. J. Schmitz et al., "Association of 25-Hydroxyvitamin D with Blood Pressure in Predominantly 25-Hydroxyvitamin D Deficient Hispanic and African Americans," *American Journal of Hypertension* 22, no. 8 (August 2009): 867–70.

21 M. D. Witham et al., "Cholecalciferol Treatment to Reduce Blood Pressure in Older Patients with Isolated Systolic Hypertension: The VitDISH Randomized Controlled Trial," *JAMA Internal Medicine* 173, no. 18 (2013): 1672–79.

22 American Heart Association, "Vitamin D Supplements May Help Blacks Lower Blood Pressure," news release, March 13, 2013, http://newsroom.heart.org/news/vitamin-d-supplements-may-help -blacks-lower-blood-pressure; and J. P. Forman et al., "Effect of Vitamin D Supplementation on Blood Pressure in Blacks," *Hypertension* 61, no. 4 (April 2013): 779–85.

23 R. B. Singh et al., "Effect of Hydrosoluble Coenzyme Q10 on Blood Pressures and Insulin Resistance in Hypertensive Patients with Coronary Artery Disease," *Journal of Human Hypertension* 13, no. 3 (March 1999): 203–8.

24 B. E. Burke, R. Neuenschwander, and R. D. Olson, "Randomized, Double-Blind, Placebo-Controlled Trial of Coenzyme Q10 in Isolated Systolic Hypertension," *Southern Medical Journal* 94, no. 11 (November 2001): 1112–17.

25 J. M. Hodgson et al., "Coenzyme Q10 Improves Blood Pressure and Glycaemic Control: A Controlled Trial in Subjects with Type 2 Diabetes," *European Journal of Clinical Nutrition* 56, no. 11 (November 2002): 1137–42.

26 MedlinePlus, "Coenzyme Q-10," www.nlm.nih.gov/medlineplus/druginfo/natural/938.html.

27 M. Wyman, M. Leonard, and T. Morledge, "Coenzyme Q10: A Therapy for Hypertension and Statin-Induced Myalgia?" *Cleveland Clinic Journal of Medicine* 77, no. 7 (July 2010): 435–42.

28 N. Sood, W. Baker, and C. Coleman, "Effect of Glucomannan on Plasma Lipid and Glucose Concentrations, Body Weight, and Blood Pressure: Systematic Review and Meta-Analysis," American Journal of Clinical Nutrition 88, no. 4 (October 2008): 1167–75.

29 NYU Langone Medical Center, "Hypertension," www.med.nyu.edu/content?ChunkIID=21725#ref38; and S. Asgary et al., "Antihypertensive and Antihyperlipidemic Effects of Achillea wilhelmsii," *Drugs under Experimental and Clinical Research* 26, no. 3 (2000): 89–93.

30 K. Kozuma et al., "Antihypertensive Effect of Green Coffee Bean Extract on Mildly Hypertensive Subjects," *Hypertension Research* 28, no. 9 (September 2005): 711–18; and NYU Department of Otolaryngology, "Green Coffee Bean Extract," http://ent.med.nyu.edu/content?ChunkIID=132201.

31 MedlinePlus, "Pycnogenol," www.nlm.nih.gov/medlineplus/druginfo/natural/1019.html.

32 Metamucil's Web site, "How a Psyllium Fiber Diet Benefits You," www.metamucil.com /psyllium-fiber-benefits.php.

33 S. Pal et al., "The Effects of 12-Week Psyllium Fibre Supplementation or Healthy Diet on Blood Pressure and Arterial Stiffness in Overweight and Obese Individuals," *British Journal of Nutrition* 107, no. 5 (March 2012): 725–34.

34 American Cancer Society, "DMSO," www.cancer.org/treatment/treatmentsandsideeffects /complementaryandalternativemedicine/pharmacologicalandbiologicaltreatment/dmso.

35 Memorial Sloan Kettering Cancer Center, "Dimethylsulfoxide," www.mskcc.org/cancer-care/herb /dimethylsulfoxide.

36 V. W. Dolinsky et al., "Resveratrol Prevents Hypertension and Cardiac Hypertrophy in Hypertensive Rats and Mice," *Biochimica et Biophysica Acta* 1832, no. 10 (October 2013): 1723–33.

37 American Heart Association, "Fish 101," www.heart.org/HEARTORG/GettingHealthy/ NutritionCenter/Fish-101/4UCM1/43059861/4Article.jsp; and F. Campbell et al., "A Systematic Review of Fish-Oil Supplements for the Prevention and Treatment of Hypertension," *European Journal of Preventive Cardiology* 20, no. 1 (February 2013): 107–20.

38 A. Basu and K. Penugonda, "Pomegranate Juice: A Heart-Healthy Fruit Juice," *Nutrition Reviews* 67, no. 1 (January 2009): 49–56.

39 C. Tsang, G. Wood, and E. Al-Dujaili, "Pomegranate Juice Consumption Influences Urinary Glucocorticoids, Attenuates Blood Pressure and Exercise-Induced Oxidative Stress in Healthy Volunteers," *Endocrine Abstracts* (2011), presented at the Society for Endocrinology BES meeting, April 2011, www.endocrine-abstracts.org/ea/0025/ea0025p139.htm.

40 MedlinePlus, "Pomegranate," www.nlm.nih.gov/medlineplus/druginfo/natural/392.html.

Chapter 16

1 American Heart Association, "Effectiveness-Based Guidelines for the Prevention of Cardiovascular Disease in Women—2011 Update," *Circulation* 123 (2011): 1243–62.

2 B. Egan et al., "Blood Pressure and Cholesterol Control in Hypertensive Hypercholesterolemic Patients: National Health and Nutrition Examination Surveys 1988–2010," *Circulation* 128 (2013): 29–41.

3 C. D. Fryar et al., "Hypertension, High Serum Total Cholesterol, and Diabetes: Racial and Ethnic Prevalence Differences in U.S. Adults, 1999–2006," *NCHS Data Brief*, no. 36 (April 2010), www.cdc.gov/nchs/data/databriefs/db36.htm.

4 Egan, "Blood Pressure and Cholesterol Control in Hypertensive Hypercholesterolemic Patients."

5 American Diabetes Association, "Treatment of Hypertension in Adults with Diabetes," *Diabetes Care* 26, no. S1 (January 2003): S80–S82.

6 CDC, "Vital Signs: Prevalence, Treatment, and Control of High Levels of Low-Density Lipoprotein Cholesterol—United States, 1999–2002 and 2005–2008," *MMWR* 60, no. 4 (February 4, 2011): 109–14.

7 E. S. Ford et al., "Hypertriglyceridemia and Its Pharmacologic Treatment among US Adults," *Archives of Internal Medicine* 169, no. 6 (March 23, 2009): 572–78.

8 C. Baigent, et al. "Efficacy and Safety of Cholesterol-Lowering Treatment: Prospective Meta-Analysis of Data from 90,056 Participants in 14 Randomised Trials of Statins," *The Lancet* 366, no. 9493 (October 8, 2005): 1267–78.

9 Preventive Cardiology Consultants, "Understanding Cholesterol," videos with transcripts, http://cvicmn.com/understandingcholesterol.php.

10 L. Mosca et al., "National Study of Women's Awareness, Preventive Action, and Barriers to Cardiovascular Health," *Circulation* 113 (2006): 525–34.

11 P. A. Huang et al., "Awareness, Accuracy, and Predictive Validity of Self-Reported Cholesterol in Women," *Journal of General Internal Medicine* 22, no. 5 (May 2007): 606–13.

12 CDC, "Vital Signs: Prevalence, Treatment, and Control."

13 P. Muntner et al., "Trends in the Prevalence, Awareness, Treatment and Control of High Low Density Lipoprotein-Cholesterol among United States Adults from 1999–2000 through 2009–2010," *American Journal of Cardiology* 112, no. 5 (September 1, 2013): 664–70.

14 M. D. Carroll, B. K. Kit, and D. A. Lacher, "Total and High-Density Lipoprotein Cholesterol in Adults: National Health and Nutrition Examination Survey, 2009–2010," *NCHS Data Brief*, no. 92 (April 2012), www.ncbi.nlm.nih.gov/pubmed/22617230.

15 Egan, "Blood Pressure and Cholesterol Control in Hypertensive Hypercholesterolemic Patients."

16 E. Powers, J. Saultz, and A. Hamilton, "Clinical Inquiries: Which Lifestyle Interventions Effectively Lower LDL Cholesterol?" *Journal of Family Practice* 56, no. 6 (June 2007): 483–85.

17 A. E. Tjonna et al., "Reversing the Metabolic Syndrome with High-Intensity Training," poster 369 at the 2006 International Symposium on Atherosclerosis, Rome, Italy, June 21, 2006, http://www.theheart.org/article/718547.do.

18 G. A. Kelley and K. S. Kelley, "Impact of Progressive Resistance Training on Lipids and Lipoproteins in Adults: A Meta-Analysis of Randomized Controlled Trials," *Preventive Medicine* 48, no. 1 (January 2009): 9–19.

19 A. Steptoe and L. Brydon, "Associations between Acute Lipid Stress Responses and Fasting Lipid Levels 3 Years Later," *Health Psychology* 24, no. 6 (November 2005): 601–7.

20 Y. Meunier, "Improving Cholesterol Profile without Drugs," presentation, http://hip.stanford.edu/online-resources/Documents/Cholesterol1/4Presentation.pdf.

21 American Diabetes Association, "Diabetes Statistics," www.diabetes.org/diabetes-basics/diabetes-statistics/.

22 A. Pan et al., "Increased Mortality Risk in Women with Depression and Diabetes Mellitus," *Archives of General Psychiatry* 68, no. 1 (January 2011): 42–50.

23 American Association of Clinical Endocrinologists, "The Burden of Prediabetes," http://outpatient.aace.com/prediabetes/the-burden-of-prediabetes.

24 L. Peeples, "'Pre-diabetes' Raises Risk of Heart Attack, Stroke," Reuters, September, 21, 2010, www.reuters.com/article/2010/09/21/us-pre-diabetes-idUSTRE68K2D320100921.

25 P. K. Crane et al., "Glucose Levels and Risk of Dementia," *New England Journal of Medicine* 369 (2013): 540–48.

26 "Diabetic Retinopathy Occurs in Pre-Diabetes," NIH News, June 12, 2005, www.nih.gov/news/pr/jun2005/niddk-12.htm.

27 C. Phend, "Kidney Disease Common in Undiagnosed and Prediabetes," *MedPage Today*, March 26, 2010, www.medpagetoday.com//Nephrology//GeneralNephrology//19236; and L. C. Plantinga et al., "Prevalence of Chronic Kidney Disease in US Adults with Undiagnosed Diabetes or Prediabetes," *Clinical Journal of the American Society of Nephrology* 5, no. 4 (April 2010): 673–82.

28 S. Dagogo-Jack, "Primary Prevention of Cardiovascular Disease in Pre-Diabetes," *Diabetes Care* 28, no. 4 (April 2005): 971–72.

29 CDC, "Prediabetes Facts," www.cdc.gov/diabetes/prevention/factsheet.htm.

30 D. A. Jenkins et al., "Effect of Legumes as Part of a Low Glycemic Index Diet on Glycemic Control

and Cardiovascular Risk Factors in Type 2 Diabetes Mellitus," *Archives of Internal Medicine* 172, no. 21 (November 26, 2012): 1653–60.

31 P. Carter et al., "Fruit and Vegetable Intake and Incidence of Type 2 Diabetes Mellitus: Systematic Review and Meta-Analysis," *British Medical Journal* 341 (August 20, 2010), doi: 10.1136/bmj.c4229.

32 E. Q. Ye et al., "Greater Whole-Grain Intake Is Associated with Lower Risk of Type 2 Diabetes, Cardiovascular Disease, and Weight Gain," *Journal of Nutrition* 142, no. 7 (July 2012): 1304–13.

33 J. A. Higgins, "Whole Grains, Legumes, and the Subsequent Meal Effect: Implications for Blood Glucose Control and the Role of Fermentation," *Journal of Nutrition and Metabolism* 2012 (2012), doi: 10.1155/2012/829238.

34 F. Zizi et al., "Sleep Duration and the Risk of Diabetes Mellitus: Epidemiologic Evidence and Pathophysiologic Insights," *Current Diabetes Reports* 10, no. 1 (February 2010): 43–47.

35 E. Donga et al., "A Single Night of Partial Sleep Deprivation Induces Insulin Resistance in Multiple Metabolic Pathways in Healthy Subjects," *Journal of Clinical Endocrinology and Metabolism* 95, no. 6 (June 2010): 2963–68.

36 Joslin Diabetes Center, "Sleep Problems and Diabetes," www.joslin.org/info/sleep1/4problems1/4and1/4diabetes.html.

37 K. L. Knutson et al., "Cross-Sectional Associations Between Measures of Sleep and Markers of Glucose Metabolism Among Subjects with and without Diabetes: The Coronary Artery Risk Development in Young Adults (CARDIA) Sleep Study," *Diabetes Care* 34, no. 5 (May 2011): 1171–76.

38 M. Hoevenaar-Blom et al., "Sufficient Sleep Duration Contributes to Lower Cardiovascular Disease Risk in Addition to Four Traditional Lifestyle Factors: The MORGEN Study," *European Journal of Preventive Cardiology*, published online July 3, 2013, www.medpagetoday.com/upload/2013/7/8/European%20Journal%20of%20Preventive%20Cardiology-2013-Hoevenaar-Blom-2047487313493057.pdf.

39 N. A. Shah et al., "Obstructive Sleep Apnea Is Associated with an Increased Risk of Coronary Artery Disease and Death," presented at the American Thoracic Society 2007 International Conference.

40 International Diabetes Federation, "Sleep Apnoea and Type 2 Diabetes," www.idf.org/sleep-apnoea-and-type-2-diabetes.

41 US Department of Health and Human Services, "Cardiovascular Diseases," chap. 6 in *How Tobacco Smoke Causes Disease: The Biology and Behavioral Basis for Smoking-Attributable Disease* (Atlanta, GA: US Department of Health & Human Services, 2010).

42 R. E. Schane et al, "Health Effects of Light and Intermittent Smoking," *Circulation* 121 (2010): 1518–22.

43 "Cardiovascular Diseases," chap. 6 in *How Tobacco Smoke Causes Disease*.

44 Ibid.

45 U. Risérus, W. C. Willett, and F. B. Hu, "Dietary Fats and Prevention of Type 2 Diabetes," *Progress in Lipid Research* 48, no. 1 (January 2009): 44–51.

46 J. C. Richards et al., "Short-Term Sprint Interval Training Increases Insulin Sensitivity in Healthy Adults but Does Not Affect the Thermogenic Response to Beta-Adrenergic Stimulation," *Journal of Physiology* 588, pt. 15 (August 1, 2010): 2961–72.

47 E. Bacchi et al., "Metabolic Effects of Aerobic Training and Resistance Training in Type 2 Diabetic Subjects," *Diabetes Care* 35, no. 4 (April 2012): 676–82.

48 S. Rosenzweig et al., "Mindfulness-Based Stress Reduction Is Associated with Improved Glycemic Control in Type 2 Diabetes Mellitus: A Pilot Study," *Alternative Therapies in Health and Medicine* 13, no. 5 (September–October 2007): 36–38.

49 L. Rasmussen-Torvik et al., "Ideal Cardiovascular Health Is Inversely Associated with Incident Cancer: The Atherosclerosis Risk in Communities Study," *Circulation* 127, no. 12 (March 2013): 1270–75.

50 E. Grossman, "Blood Pressure: The Lower, the Better," supplement, *Diabetes Care* 34, no. S2 (May 2011): S308–S312.

Chapter 17

1 J. Hollis et al., "Weight Loss During the Intensive Intervention Phase of the Weight-Loss Maintenance Trial," *American Journal of Preventive Medicine* 35, no. 2 (August 2008): 118–26.

Index

Underscored page references indicate sidebars and tables. **Boldface** references indicate photographs.